I'M ALRIGHT

Overcoming Physical and

Emotional Abuse Through Faith

James G. Jones, MD

I have tried to recreate events, locales and conversations from my memories. In some instances, I have changed the names of individuals and places, to maintain their anonymity and protect their privacy. I may also have changed some identifying characteristics and details such as physical properties, occupations and places of residence.

Dedication

I'm alright is dedicated to the memory of Courtland F. Kanzinger. The man who inspired me to dream big. And to my dear friend Ed Whitaker. Ed saw this book before I wrote it. And to my daughter Onycha, who inspired me to fall in love with books again. You all served as the wind beneath my wings.

CONTENTS

INTRODUCTION

My Purpose

I clasp my trembling hands as I look through a cracked dusty window up to the heavens. I blink to stop the sting of salty tears as they stream down my face. My back and legs throb from the fresh still bleeding welts. The welts are a result of the lash of an extension cord less than twelve hours ago. I feel fear from the top of my head down to my toes. Fear flows to every organ, every cell and every atom of my body. I look heavenward for relief. I fear another beating is forthcoming. My six-year-old body cannot take another beating. Truth is, my psyche can't take another assault.

I felt I would lose my mind if I had to endure another beating. My only crime was that I had put a few morsels of food in my pocket and retreated to my third floor bedroom, the only place in my childhood home where I could enjoy it. I was afforded very few pleasures as a child in Philadelphia. I grew up in a house, ruthlessly controlled by my Gene, my mother's paramour whom we called our stepfather. My childhood home was a place that was full of chaos and emotional turmoil. Gene was responsible for the wounds and scars on my body. He was the cause of my fear. One of my brothers, Carl, saw me nibbling on a biscuit I had stuffed in my pocket. Carl said he was going to tell Gene despite my begging him not to do so. My stepfather was never one to use words, instead he preferred to let extension cords speak for him. I couldn't endure that kind of conversation; I was on my knees seeking divine intervention.

I felt that all was lost in that moment until I remembered Jesus. My mother used to take us to church when we lived in Newark, NJ, and I knew He could help me. I prayed fervently in that moment as I heard my brother run down the steps to tell Gene what I had done. I prayed for Jesus to intervene. He did. My stepfather did not act on my brother's disclosure.

This moment stands out in my memory as I look over the story of my life. While I had to endure multiple beatings after that, there was never a moment when things were so dire. It was rare for me to have a measure of hope in my childhood. As time passed subsequent beatings and verbal assaults snatched away the hope I tried to fervently hold on to. Childhood turmoil laid the foundation for a tumultuous adulthood. My life would be plagued with many difficulties.

Difficulties in life have a way of thrusting you toward your destiny. I could never have thought that I would write a book about the adversities I experienced in my life. Yet here I am about to embark on a journey that has been healing for me. It is my hope that sharing my story will lead you to your own healing. As an adult, I have had to cope with what, at times, seemed to be the fickle nature of life. I often wondered what was driving the decisions I made. I had always thought I had good intentions when I made these decisions. Although my intentions appeared at the time to be good, as I look back I see that many of my decisions have had a devastating impact on my life. I'm writing *I'm Alright* as I am going through my second divorce. How did I get here? How can I make sense of this? It would have been so easy to blame others or a set of circumstances to account for my predicament. As easy as it would be to blame others for the negative outcomes I have faced, I had to admit the truth, what these circumstances all have in common, is me. I knew that to make sense of my life I had to find the answer within myself. Thus, began my journey to find the motivation for my decisions.

It was an amazing feeling when I started this existential quest. I could never have imagined that it would include writing a book. I needed to share my journey from denial to acceptance of myself. I tended to look at the parts of myself that I was willing to accept and to ignore the parts I found unacceptable. In order to be whole, I needed to accept all of me, warts and all. I initially viewed myself as a victim of childhood trauma. Now, I view myself as a survivor of the abuse that gnawed at my very soul. My trauma transformed me from a free-spirited child who wore a sunny smile to a fretful child who grew into a broken shell of a man. Although early in my adult life I was conscious of some of the impact that my childhood experience had on me, it wasn't until later that I became aware of the full impact. I see how my unconscious struggles have manifested into a web of chaos that ensnared me and refused to let go.

I often viewed various disappointing events as disparate entities. I now see the patterns. I consciously recreated the chaos that I endured during my childhood. With each stumble, I now see how I slowly slid into the abyss of despair. Writing this book has been a purifying experience. In expressing my truth, I had to be vulnerable. In that vulnerable state, I sought desperately to look inward to find a solution. During college, I sought therapy. My therapist initially diagnosed me with dysthymia, a mild form of depression, and then Major Depression, a more severe form of depression. Traditional talk therapy and medication alleviated some of my symptoms but not all. The despair that gnawed at my soul never went away. I met with many other well-meaning therapists but they missed the mark. I believe my search for the truth lead me to a career in psychiatry after graduating from Temple University School of Medicine. Searching for answers, I expanded my psychiatric knowledge. Great clinical supervision helped to provide me with appropriate context for that knowledge. I also continued individual therapy, but I was disappointed because despondency was ever present. I yearned for relief.

I used to concern myself with what others thought of me. I tried to hide my past as if it was something to be embarrassed of. But my past would eventually push me to accept my truth and allow that truth to shine. I realize that some people may choose to ridicule me because of my disclosures. Those that do are not my audience. They are not who I am trying to reach. They are like my inner critic, which for years, sought to control me with the cold claws of consternation. I am trying to reach those who are survivors of abuse, or who are currently experiencing abuse. They are my audience. It is through my vulnerability that I may be able to reach them. If I have described you, please read on as I take you on a journey from the lost innocence of childhood to the triumph of the indomitable human spirit.

I want to be clear as I discuss the events of my life, who has been most helpful through this journey. It is my Lord and Savior Jesus Christ. I am not a theologian, nor am I a pastor. I am simply a sinner saved by grace. I do not enter this trek believing in my own ability. I know I am guided by Him. Jesus uses me as well as other psychiatrists, psychologists, psychotherapists, treatment modalities, and medication. God allows the use of alternative approaches such as yoga and meditation as well. He has created everything in this world and has given many wonderful individuals the opportunity to serve His children whether these individuals are believers or not. In times of struggle I am always reminded of my favorite bible verse Romans 8:28 (KJV), "And we know all things work together for good for them that love God, to them who are called according to His purpose."

I am overwhelmed and honored that God, in His infinite wisdom has decided to use me to point others in His direction. Jesus is that ray of light that will shine into the chasm of despair many survivors of childhood abuse find themselves in. He is the Way, the Truth and the Life. I pray that you will find that I have been faithful to what He asked me to do.

Not long ago, I had a conversation with a dear longtime friend of mine, Ed Whitaker. I first met him shortly after completing my psychiatry residency at Temple University Hospital. One of my responsibilities as a newly minted psychiatry attending was to serve as an expert witness at a civil mental health court hearing. As a psychiatrist-in-training, I was not qualified to testify, but after completing my training in 1996, suddenly I was. On the day I met Ed, I did not feel prepared for that seemingly daunting responsibility. I was dressed in an ill-fitting black pinstriped suit. I guess Ed could tell that I was nervous. The beads of sweat on my forehead must have betrayed my façade of confidence. He helped me get through that harrowing day and he has been supportive of me ever since. A few years ago, he told me I should write a book. At that time, I thought it was odd since I had never written one. I also didn't think I had a book in me. After more recent life events, I am now compelled to write one. On a spring day in 2015, while sitting on a comfy couch in the family room of Ed's home, I told him I had started to write that book. I told him I had many starts and stops. Ed told me to write from my heart and the words would flow, so here goes.

The title of my book is *I'm Alright*. "I'm alright" is a common phrase used to respond to the question, how are you? It is a benign response often given as a verbal reflex. It is often used to portray a sense of normalcy. The reality is that most of the time, the person asking the question is simply being polite and doesn't expect a real answer, so the stock response of I'm alright is easily accepted. Depending on their relationship the person answering often does not respond truthfully as to not reveal troubling issues to an acquaintance. My purpose in writing I'm *Alright* is not to ask the reason for the question but rather to delve into the sometimes-automatic response to it.

There may be several reasons to explain why the answer is often "I'm alright". One reason may be to avoid discussing the pain of deep dark secrets from our past. We worry about what others would think about us if they knew our issues. Maybe we want to maintain the mask we wear to hide our pain. Perhaps like me, you wanted to portray a sense of normalcy. I wanted to hold on to a false reality of my childhood; one I believed should have been bursting with happiness. I wanted a childhood filled with magical thinking and untold joy, where visions of sugar plums danced in my head. I wanted fond memories of birthdays and Christmas gifts, of wonderful family vacations and get-togethers. At least that's want I saw in the eyes of my classmates and on television. It was with this imaginary context that I created my veneer of normality. Truth was this was never my reality. My childhood was filled with fear and pain. I am a survivor of horrific childhood abuse.

As a survivor of such abuse there is guilt and shame that reached to the core of my being. I learned to adapt by wearing a mask of normalcy despite feeling like I didn't quite fit in. Shame prevented me from sharing my true feelings. How can you put into words the enormity of such pain; the pain of being hurt by people who should have protected you? Every organ of my body ached. The very atoms of my being are bathed in a fire of suffering. As much as I tried to run away from it, my past always caught up to me.

My purpose in writing this is to share my journey. In doing so I hope it creates a dialogue among childhood abuse survivors to find their own voice. In my pain, I responded to the question, "how are you?" by saying, "I'm alright" even though I wasn't. What I felt on the inside was that I was a failure, that I was stupid. How can I tell anyone that I thought I was a terrible father even though I have children who love me? Despite completing graduate school and earning a good living, I am drowning in debt. Even though I desire the company of people who love and care about me, I am uncomfortable around them and often feel alone in a crowd of people. Yet when I am alone I crave company. I look at other people and they seem so happy and I felt so miserable.

I felt the need to don a mask of normalcy even though my innermost feelings betray me, especially when I looked in a mirror. I would see the sadness that had been in my eyes for far too long. That is the main reason that in the past I seldom made eye contact. I felt so sad because of my childhood. The burden of those secrets kept me captive. I know that I must shed the burden of my past, but it is not enough for me to do it alone. I must share my journey with other survivors of abuse to encourage them to do the same.

I will not carry the weight of guilt and shame into this new season of my life. It was important for me to say I was alright back then even though I didn't feel that way so I could feel accepted. The truth was I felt broken. It was strange to me that no one even noticed how broken I was. I felt like an alien trapped in a world of happy people. Everyone seemed so happy and content with their lives. When I looked in the mirror into my eyes, I saw despair but I was too ashamed to talk about it. How could I burden anyone with my misery? As a child, I learned that no one cared so what was the purpose of talking to anyone or trying to change anything. I had even convinced myself to ignore those thoughts until vestiges of my past would ooze out in the form of feelings of insecurity and a need for constant validation.

As a child, I had to endure horrific emotional abuse and neglect by my mother and stepfather, as well as horrendous physical abuse by my stepfather. I was also neglected by my aunts and uncles, whom I later found out were aware of my abuse but did nothing. As an adult, my past shaped my behavior. I became an adulterer. I had a child out of wedlock. I divorced my first wife with little to no regard as to how this would hurt our children. Hurt people hurt people. Afterward, I would berate myself for being the selfish man that my biological father was.

I mismanaged my finances and lost my home to foreclosure. My credit rating plummeted. None of this is a secret to those who know me. I choose to share this with you because I am stepping out of the shadow of my shame. I can no longer let my past control me as I walk toward the light of my healing. It's as if I am pregnant with the burden of my abuse. I am going through psychological labor pain. I am afraid of the unknown. Still I must go on. I am about to give birth to the new me.

I must accept my current reality. I must also seek to understand how it is connected to my past. I must embrace my reality in the present. I must feel the warmth of the sun today and not be haunted by the chill of the past. I must taste the sweet nectar of the now and not the bitter pill of days gone by. The mellifluous tones of the present are far more grounding than the cacophony of my chaotic past. Each day I face the struggle of staying ever present and grounded in the here and now, in this moment; but it is worth it. I have endured a lot. I am truly a survivor.

In this book, I hope to connect with other survivors. Together we can step into today and walk into a balanced and healthy future for we are survivors not victims of our past experiences. While it can sometimes be painful to look at our past, it is helpful to do so to reprocess feelings that were never dealt with at a time when we were most vulnerable. I want to start a process that should be completed with the development of a strong support system. My support system is comprised of a skilled therapist, my religious community, and a close group of dear friends. Yours may include the same. I include my family as well. For some of you, family may not be an option initially. In some cases, your family may have been the source of abuse. In those situations, a new *therapeutic* family is important. That is not to say that anyone should give up on their family because of past abuse. As you work through your therapeutic process and achieve your healing, you can reach back and help your family heal with the support of your therapeutic family. In doing so you become the seed of hope your family needs. The flower of your growth will uproot the weeds of misery and despair in your family. You can become the fruit of forgiveness.

I have changed the names of my stepfather, my siblings and my first and second wife. I want to protect their privacy, but mostly I want to keep the focus on me. I want to explain my experience without casting aspersions on anyone. I think that blame, can hinder recovery and healing from childhood abuse. As a child, I had to cope with my trauma with the resources I had available. My task at that time was simply to survive. Those experiences impacted my development. I am solely responsible for my actions as an adult. I am responsible for how my actions affected my relationships. In that light, I believe that it is far more important that I not mention the names of people who have been negatively impacted by my actions. I can reveal my struggles without causing undue pain to others.

About Me

I am a fifty-five-year-old Christian African-American psychiatrist. I believe I am my father's third of six children. I was told that my biological father was an alcoholic. I never actually saw him intoxicated or even drink alcohol. That may because he was not involved in my life. Perhaps he didn't want me to see that part of him. I am my mother's second child of her six children. Although both of my parents had six children, each had two children from other relationships. My parents were married sometime before I started school. Family legend has it that when my mother was pregnant with me, her second child, but her first with my father, he denied that I was his. I was given the name Gregory Burton Hall at the time of my birth. My aunts and uncles called me Burt. I didn't find this out why until I was a teenager. I always wondered why everyone called me Burt when my name was James Gregory Jones. I now understand.

I have no memories of my parents being together, and no memories of a happy family. I guess that was not God's plan for me. I have been in pursuit of that mythical family all my life. Even as a young child I latched onto any family that would have me. I felt that being a part of a family would provide me the comfort I was missing. I wanted to be part of something bigger than myself.

In the telling of my story it is important to give you appropriate context. It is important to understand the context of my life to fully understand my process. To that end, I will divide the circumstances of my journey in the following manner. First I will talk about how psychiatry has impacted African-American history. I will then talk about how I transitioned from a happy child into an abused child who was wracked with fear. Next, I will discuss my journey into psychiatry. Finally, I will outline how these issues culminate into a better understanding of myself. Throughout my journey, I will talk about how my Christian faith matured.

PSYCHIATRY AND AFRICAN-AMERICAN CULTURE

To understand my journey, it was important for me to see mental health through the lens of the African-American experience. I remember as a young child, hearing the adults talk about someone having a nervous breakdown. As an inquisitive kid, I asked what that was, but I was never given a clear answer. Mental illness was not a topic that was openly discussed in my household or those of my friends. I recall straining to hear what was said after the adults mentioned someone had a nervous breakdown. Often what followed was hushed whispers as I was ushered out of the room. There was always a shroud of mystery when my family would have those conversations as if there was a sense of shame.

As I read about the impact psychiatry had on the African American experience, I was beginning to understand why this was the case. As with Christianity, which I'll discuss later, psychiatry was used to the detriment of the African diaspora. As the agrarian economy in the United States began to grow, a cheap source of labor was needed. Native Americans were first used as slaves but that was not a successful venture. Soon Africans were taken captive and brought to the United States. As Africans were captured and enslaved, they were separated from their homeland and their way of life. Their language, culture and heritage and history was ripped from them. Over the course of generations of enslavement, they lost the soul of who they were and where they came from. My ancestors were trapped in a society that narcissistically thought their African culture was inferior. Without understanding the enslaved Africans, early American psychiatrists attempted to turn a slave's very human desire to be free into pathology.

Vanessa Jackson in her excellent paper, *In Our Own Voice*, demonstrates how psychiatry and mental health systems have had a detrimental impact on the psyche of African-Americans. She provides insight into the ugly side of psychiatry. It a side of psychiatry that should not be ignored because those events have repercussions today, even though most African-Americans are not aware of them.

Benjamin Rush MD, a face of early American psychiatry and one of the founding fathers of the United States of America, described a condition called Negritude. He said it was a disease that affected American Negroes. He thought that Negritude was a mild form of leprosy. The only cure for this disorder he proposed was for the American Negro to become white. It was unclear whether anyone was successfully cured from the disorder. Despite holding this opinion, Dr. Rush was a leading voice in reforming mental health treatment and was involved in the anti-slavery movement.

In 1851, Dr. Samuel Cartwright, a Louisiana physician, published "Report On The Diseases and Physical Peculiarities of the Negro Race" in *The New Orleans Medical and Surgical Journal*. In that paper, Dr. Cartwright wrote that he discovered two diseases to the American Negro which justified their enslavement. He first described drapetomania, which he stated caused Negroes to run away because of mania or craziness. Dr. Cartwright asserted that any slave who demonstrated dissatisfied behavior should be whipped severely as an early intervention. He noted that overseers should be vigilant for evidence of drapetomania. He believed that slaves should be made to be submissive and encouraged to be in a childlike state. He also contradicted himself by stating that it would take "care, kindness, attention, and humanity, to prevent and cure them from running away." It is hard to imagine how anyone capable of severely whipping anyone can then demonstrate compassion.

Dr. Cartwright also diagnosed slaves with Dyaesthesia Aethiopica or "hebetude of the mind and obtuse sensibility of the body—a disease peculiar to Negroes called—Rascality." What made Dyaethesia Aethiopica different from other mental disorders was the physical signs and lesions associated with it. Dr. Cartwright also stated that whipping was the treatment for Dyaesthesia Aethiopica. One must wonder if previous whippings were the true cause of the lesions he associated with Dyaesthesia Aethiopica.

Dr. Cartwright was a leading thinker in the pro-slavery movement and challenged the anti-slavery movement. Dr. Cartwright also wrote, "Diseases and Peculiarities of the Negro Race." In that article, he admonished his opposition by stating, "The northern physician and people have noticed the symptoms, but not the disease from which they spring. They ignorantly attribute the symptoms to the debasing influence of slavery on the mind without considering that those who have never been in slavery, or their fathers before them, are the most afflicted, and the latest from the slave-holding south the least. The disease is the natural offspring of Negro liberty—the liberty to be idle, to wallow in filth, and to indulge in improper food and drinks."

Although written with the intent to provide a scientific explanation for the behaviors of my ancestors, one cannot avoid the clear biases Dr. Cartwright held. Early in his article, he mentions that, "If the white man attempts to oppose the Deity's will, by trying to make the negro anything else than 'the submissive knee bender,' (which the Almighty declared he should be) by trying to raise him to the level with himself, or by putting himself on an equality with the negro; or if he abuses the power which God has given him over his fellow man..." He further writes, "but if he keeps him (the negro) in the position that we learn from the Scriptures he was intended to occupy, that is, the position of submission...) Clearly, he was twisting scripture to fit his agenda for there is nothing in the bible that supports his assertions.

It is dangerous to read scriptures and cite them out of context, as many far more qualified than I would attest. If you have an agenda, you might be able to twist the Holy Bible to make a point. That is why context is so important. In the discussion of the submission of the slaves in the Bible 1 Peter 2:18-25(KJV) states, "servants should submit to their masters as a way of suffering as Christ did." Ephesians 6:5-9(KJV), also made this point. Ephesians 6:8 specifically encouraged servants to submit to their masters, "knowing that whatsoever good thing that a man doeth, the same shall he receive of the Lord. Ephesians 6:9(KJV) encouraged masters to be kind to their servant by stating, "And ye masters, do the same thing unto them, forbearing threatening: knowing that your Master also is in heaven; neither is there a respect of persons with him." Most importantly the Holy Bible states in Mark 12:31(KJV), "…. Thou shalt love thy neighbor as thyself. There is none other commandment greater than these."

Certainly, if Dr. Cartwright used the Holy Bible as it was intended by God, he would have discovered that the entire book discusses our need for Jesus Christ. In the Old Testament, God shows us that through Israel, we could not completely follow God's law no matter how hard we tried. Time and time again Israel failed. The Old Testament demonstrated that Israel needed a Savior who came in the form of Jesus Christ, who was God who took human form. Jesus suffered and died for the sins of Israel and for all who believed in Him. Slaves were focused on the long suffering of Jesus. His suffering resonated with theirs. Despite His suffering, Christ's concern and love helped them to endure the sheer brutality of slavery. That is the indomitable spirit of many African Americans today.

On the other side of the equations, many of the slave owners, like Dr. Cartwright used the Holy Bible to control what they thought was a defeated disillusioned and uneducated people. Clearly, he ignored two important points. First of all, the very words of the Bible demanded that the slave owners treat the slaves much more humanely than they were. Most importantly, the pro-slavery movement underestimated how through the power of God, the faith and commitment of the slaves, the abolitionist, and Americans opposed to slavery, helped to ensure its demise. Ironically, the very

Bible Dr. Cartwright used to justify slavery helped to defeat slavery and many who sought to justify it.

It is hard to understand how Dr. Cartwright and those involved in the pro-slavery movement could harbor so much animosity toward slaves. To them the slaves were less than human. I am reminded of a passage from C. S. Lewis' book, *Mere Christianity*. In his book, he states how this hatred is developed when he discussed how the Germans could be so cruel to the Jewish people. He wrote, "The Germans, perhaps, at first ill-treated the Jews because they hated them: afterwards they hated them much more because they had ill-treated them. The crueler you are, the more you will hate: and the more you hate, the crueler you will become—and so on in a vicious circle forever."

His words resonated with me. It gave me a window into mindset of how so many people could have been so cruel. Their vicious attacks were committed verbally, physically and culturally. My ancestors were no longer seen as fully human. This point was clearly made at the 1787 United States Constitutional Convention where a compromise was reached between delegates from southern states and northern states to determine a state's population for legislative representation. It was determined that slave would be counted as three-fifths of a person. This is one of the reasons why it was so difficult for my ancestors to be seen as and treated as human.

There are countless books documenting the cruelty encountered by slaves. In Chapter 4 of her book, *Post Traumatic Slave Syndrome,* Dr. Joy DeGruy documents the writings of then former slave Henry Bibb (1949).

"Who can imagine what could be the feelings of a father and mother, when looking upon their infant child whipped and tortured with impunity, and placed in a situation where they could afford it no protection. But we were all claimed and held as property; the father and the mother were slaves... I was compelled to stand and see my wife shamefully scourged and abused by her master: and the manner in which this was done, was so violently and inhumanely committed upon the person of a female, that I despair in finding decent language to describe the bloody act of cruelty. My happiness or pleasure was then all blasted; for it was sometimes a pleasure to be with my family even in slavery. I loved them as my wife and child. Little Francis was a pretty child; she was quiet, playful, bright, and interesting. But I could never look upon the dear child without being filled with sorrow and fearful apprehensions of being separated by slave holders, because she was a slave, regarded as property. And unfortunately for me, I am the father of a slave… It calls fresh to my mind the separation of husband and wife: of stripping, tying up and flogging; of tearing children from their parents, and selling them on the auction block. It calls to mind female virtue, virtue trampled underfoot.

But oh! When I remember that my daughter, my only child, is still there, destined to share the fate of all these calamities, it is too much to bear… If ever there was any one act of my life while a slave, that I have to lament over, it is that of being a father and a husband of slaves."

Frederick Douglass wrote in his book *My Bondage, My Freedom*, about what he and others endured as slaves. He wrote about a slave named Demby. Mr. Douglass wrote "…I knew him well. He was a powerful young man, full of animal spirits, and, as far as I know, he was among the most valuable of Col. Lloyd's slaves. In something—I know not what—he offended Mr. Austin Gore (the overseer), and in accordance with the custom of the latter, he undertook to flog him. He gave Denby (Demby) but few stripes; the latter broke away from him and plunged into a creek, and then standing there to the depth of his neck in the water, he refused to come out at the order of the overseer; whereupon, for this refusal Gore shot him dead!"

Mr. Douglass states that the overseer's action was predicated on the cruel notion that all affronts by slaves must be met with force, which could end in murder and those who acted did so with impunity.

It is so sad to think of how my ancestors, in their pursuit of happiness away from the grips of horrific slavery, were deemed pathological by the prominent psychiatrist of that time. It is equally sad that the idea that to whip the slaves would be appropriate treatment for nonexistent mental illnesses. Untold millions of slaves were severely beaten, some killed in the process. Any clear minded person who was faced by that brutality would indeed try to escape. Dr. Cartwright, and many similar minded individuals, ignore the brutality, the squalor and the powerlessness that slaves had to endure. Slaves sought the freedom and the opportunity to be self-determined and not under the control of people who did not have their best interest at heart. I consider their pursuit of freedom, normal, healthy and not at all pathological.

Slaves earned their freedom via the Emancipation Proclamation, which was an executive order by Abraham Lincoln on January 1, 1863. This proclamation changed the status of my ancestors from slaves to free people. Its impact was not immediately felt by the slaves because many southern slave holders refused to inform them. Many slaves who fled to the North were amazed to learn on their arrival that they had no fear of being returned for they were free. Unfortunately, this didn't stop American psychiatrists from looking at the newly freed slaves through the lens of their bigotry. In 1895, Dr. Theophilus O. Powell, superintendent of the Georgia Lunatic Asylum and a renowned scholar in psychiatry, noted what he thought was an alarming increase in insanity by the Negroes in Georgia. He asserted that this level of mental illness was unheard of prior to 1860.

Census records between 1860 and 1890 showed that mental illness in Negroes had increased from 1 in 10,584 to 1 in 943. Dr. Powell theorized that hygienic and structured lives led by the slaves served as a protective measure against insanity. Dr. Powell stated,

"Freedom, however, removed all hygienic restraints, and they were no longer obedient to the inexorable laws of health, plunging into all sort of excesses and vices, leading irregular lives, and having apparently little or no control over their appetites and passions." He basically said that freedom made my ancestors mentally ill. The implication was that slaves needed the care of slave holders to tend to their every need.

This is of course far from the truth. This truth, however, was ignored in favor of looking for mental illness in many of the newly free slaves were there was none. Many involved in the pro-slavery movement used Dr. Powell's rhetoric to bolster their position. Many of them pointed to the 1840 United States census, which showed an increase in mental illness among free Negroes. African-American physician, Dr. James McCune Smith argued against the 1840 census. He wrote, "Freedom has not made us mad. It strengthened our minds by throwing us upon our own resources." Other factors that could have led to the manifestation of mental illness in the slaves during the post-Civil War era were starvation and poor nutrition that lead to vitamin deficiencies. Disease as a result of poor nutrition affected displaced former slaves.

Many of the newly freed slaves in the South were held as though they were imprisoned in lunatic asylums. The Georgia Lunatic Asylum was, at that time, the largest in the world. It was initially operated with the use of slave labor. In his book, *Mad in America: Bad Science, Bad Medicine and the Enduring Mistreatment of the Mentally Ill* Robert Whitaker writes on page 171: "After the Civil War ended, Southern Negroes, emancipated from their bonds of slavery, found themselves newly at risk of being locked up in mental asylums. The definition of sanity in Negroes was still tied to behavior that a slave owner liked to see: a docile, hardworking laborer who paid him proper respect. Negroes who strayed too far from that behavioral norm were candidates for being declared insane and were put away in asylums, jails and poorhouses."

Lynn Gamwell and Nancy Tomes wrote in their book, *Madness in America: Cultural and Medical Perceptions of Mental Illness before 1914*, (Page 56): "Because the number of free Blacks in the North was relatively small, northern asylums had few African-American applicants. Some private asylums, including Friends

Asylum (in Philadelphia), simply did not admit Blacks. While others, like Pennsylvania Hospital for the Insane, discreetly kept quiet about its admissions. State mental hospitals accepted African Americans more openly but placed them in segregated wards or separate buildings where they had fewer amenities than White patients. Most commonly, public officials assumed that the expense of hospital treatment was wasted on Blacks, who were confined instead in jails and almshouses, where they received decidedly inferior care."   In Vanessa Jackson's *"Separate and Unequal: The Legacy of Racially Segregated Psychiatric Hospitals A Cultural Competence Training Tool,"* she cites an excerpt from *Working Cures: Healing Health and Power on Southern Slave Plantation* by Sharla M. Fett which documents a history of medical abuse and neglect of African Americans from enslavement to the present time. The introduction notes: "White physicians and medical students subjected enslaved men and women to experimentation and humiliating displays as medical specimens. By the late nineteenth century, white pundits and scientist alike employed evolutionary theory and population statistics to project the extinction of the 'Negro race.' Twentieth century eugenics forced sterilization of poor women, nonconsensual experimentation and massive discrimination complete a history of medical abuse built on a legacy of slavery and racism. This historical accounting clearly renders African American distrust of white medical institution, to borrow sociologist Kirk Johnson's phrase, 'a sensible act.'"

It comes as no surprise that African-Americans continue to not trust the institution of American medicine and psychiatry. Given the history of slavery and how it cast a distorted view of African-Americans in the eyes of Americans of European descent, who represent most the population and who continue to wield enormous cultural, political and financial power. African-Americans often feel that they must continually guard against being treated as second-class citizens.

The disconnect between American psychiatry and the African-American experience reemerged during the Civil Rights era. African Americans asserted their desire for equal treatment under the law in a more forceful manner. The decision to protest for those rights were not without significant risks. Much has been made of the efforts of Dr. Martin Luther King, Malcolm X, and Huey P. Newton and many others. They were rightfully lauded for their commitment to uplift the lives of African-Americans. Their contributions are remarkable. I am also amazed by the dedication of the African-American citizens who placed themselves in harm's way. They were subjected to verbal taunts, physical assaults, and were even murdered. They were so committed to their cause that they were willing to risk their lives. They were heroic in their own right.

Instead of viewing the actions of African Americans as courageous, it was considered pathological. In 1968, psychiatrists Dr. Walter Bromberg and Dr. Franck Simon co-authored an article in the *Archives of General Psychiatry* titled "The 'Protest' Psychosis." In it the actions of Civil Rights protestors were viewed a result of pathology, as a form of schizophrenia. This is like the discussions African descendants during slavery, when their desire to be treated in a humane fashion was seen as pathological, the actions of those seeking civil rights were considered a sign of mental illness. The article showed that American psychiatry continued to be blind to our humanity. It was far more important for American psychiatry to maintain the status quo rather than consider the anguished eyes of the civil rights protestors. The paper was influential in regarding how schizophrenia was diagnosed in the United States of America.

In the book, *The Protest Psychosis: How Schizophrenia Became a Black Disease,* Jonathan M. Metzl discuss how prior to this article, schizophrenia was thought to be a rare disorder associated with middle-class housewives who were associated with nonthreatening behavior. They were encouraged to be nurtured by their psychiatrist. It was popular between the 1920s and the1950s to depict schizophrenics erroneously as a psychoanalytic condition of these housewives. Many researchers would perform their studies on Caucasian only wards. Schizophrenics of different racial backgrounds were largely ignored and rendered invisible. The American view of schizophrenia began to change in the 1960s as race, gender and temperament were now taken into consideration. The shift was away from the idea that schizophrenics were docile, to considering them to be people full of rage. Psychiatric journals began to note this rageful behavior in "Negro men."

I would be remiss if I didn't discuss the role prominent psychiatrists of African descent have had on mental health treatment. *Black Psychiatrist and American Psychiatry,* published by the American Psychiatric Association and edited by Jeanne Spurlock, MD is a great resource. Dr. Solomon Carter Fuller, who was born in

Liberia, received his medical education from Boston University in 1897. He is credited as the first Black psychiatrist. Dr. Fuller received his psychiatric training at Boston University. After completing his training, he sought a position in psychiatry in the United States but was unable to find one. He decided to pursue a position abroad. In Europe, he received additional training under Dr. Emil Kraepein among others, at the University of Munich. After completing his additional training, he returned to the United States where he became a clinician, researcher, and neurologist at Westborough State Hospital and remained there for forty-five years.

Another prominent Black psychiatrist was Dr. Charles Prudhomme. Dr. Prudhomme graduated from Howard University School of Medicine in 1935. He applied for but was not accepted for formal training in psychiatry at Saint Elizabeth's Hospital. He then worked at Tuskegee VA Hospital as a medical director. Dr. Prudhomme completed psychoanalytic training at the Washington Psychoanalytic Institute in 1956. He is said to be the first Black-American psychoanalyst and was often the victim of racist practices. Dr. Prudhomme became an activist and was influential in the desegregation of VA hospitals. He was also involved in the landmark case Brown v. Board of Education of Topeka, Kansas (1954). During that time, Dr. Prudhomme approached the American Psychiatric Association for their support for the desegregation of schools. He did not receive their support and was encourage to avoid involvement in such a political issue. He did not listen to them.

In Philadelphia, PA we were blessed by the pioneering work of African-American psychiatrist Dr. Warren Edward Smith. In 1954, he graduated with honors from the pre-med program at LaSalle College. He attended Hahnemann Medical College in 1957. He began a practice in general medicine in the West Oak Lane section of Philadelphia. Dr. Smith became fascinated with the connection between the mental health and medical issues of his patients. He decided to pursue a career in psychiatry and entered formal training at Albert Einstein Medical Center and the Hahnemann Hospital. He became a consultant to the Philadelphia School District, Archdiocesan Schools and the Baptist Children's Home. He also taught Philadelphia police officers how to recognize signs of mental illness. He was one of the founding members of the Earlene Houston Psychiatric Society, which consists of a group of African-American psychiatrists who encourage African-American physicians to pursue a career in psychiatry. He has had a tremendous influence on several African-American psychiatrists in Philadelphia as a colleague, mentor and role model.

The focus on emphasizing cultural competence helped the field of mental health to acknowledge the importance of understanding people from various ethnic backgrounds. In 2006, the state of California passed Assembly Bill 1195. This bill required that continuing medical education provide content on cultural and linguistic competency. In this way, physicians would be able to maintain the professional development to treat an ever-changing demographic. For African Americans, and other ethnic groups, this meant that finally cultural context would be taken under consideration when decisions regarding medical and mental health issues are addressed. This would also allow for mutual consideration between care providers and recipients in a culturally sensitive manner that was not available before.

Joy DeGruy, PhD. In her book *Post Traumatic Slave Syndrome*, talks about the lingering impact slavery has had on the African-American culture. Dr. DeGruy gives a vivid illustration of the detrimental effects oppression can have on a people in Chapter 4 of her book, she recounts a visit to South African village of Ndebele in 1994. As she sat in the living room she observed in a corner, ten or twelve children huddled together. Their ages ranged from toddlers to young teens. She remarked about how well they played together; they were seen but barely heard. She was amazed how ecstatic they were to be in the presence of an African-American woman. Dr. DeGruy was also amazed how these children had such a clear understanding of their role in the family system.

She later visited another village in South Africa called Onverwagt, which in Afrikaans means "unexpected." The inhabitants of this village were the descendants of Africans who were once enslaved by the Dutch. After Apartheid ended, they represented a blight on South African History. Dr. DeGruy was escorted through the village by a middle-aged couple who were committed to helping the people of Onverwagt, many of whom were practically starving to death.

These two villages were markedly different. The people from Onverwagt had no tribal affiliations, in contrast, the people of Ndebele maintained tribal associations. The people of Onverwagt had no tribal language or culture, something that the Ndebele maintained. The people of Onverwagt held on to names they received from their former slave owners and relied heavily on the Afrikaans culture that enslaved them, but did not claim them.

In observing the people of the Onverwagt, Dr. DeGruy felt that she had a glimpse into what must have been the experience of the antebellum South. The people of Onverwagt wore clothing similar to southern sharecroppers. Their self-esteem was shattered. They walked around with their heads lowered and averted direct eye contact. They were plagued with drug and alcohol abuse, domestic violence and crime. They carried the unyielding burden of feelings of low self-esteem and low self-worth. This was in marked contrast to the Ndebele children who, although equally poor, had a sense of well-being and possessed a gentle nature that the Onverwagt did not. That contrast can be seen today in the African diaspora and in native Africans.

The realization of the sheer brutality of slavery encoded in the collective unconscious of African Americans today, helps me to understand what a nervous breakdown is. It is the stirring of the soul that starts as a low level of fear that quickly reaches a crescendo. It is the guttural release of deep seated emotional pain that can no longer be contained or denied. It is the release of inner unconscious turmoil that percolates to the surface of consciousness. It is frightening to those who experience this type of suffering and to those who provide comfort. It is this reason why the adults in my family sheltered young children from witnessing it, because it would be both difficult to explain and equally difficult for a child to understand.

NEWARK BURT

My journey into healing began with memories. They were memories that I struggled with, and those that I wanted to forget but couldn't. Along the way, I had to remember that all of my memories were not filled with dread. The fond memories make me smile. I recall a scene from the 1986 award-winning television movie

Promise. It starred James Garner as, Bobby, who promised his dying mother that he would take care of his schizophrenic younger brother DJ, who was movingly portrayed by James Woods.

In a poignant scene, Bobby, in hopes of breaking DJ out of his daily pattern of isolating himself at home watching television and chain smoking, implores him to go on a fishing trip. DJ finally agrees. They drive to a remote cabin where they'd stayed in the past when they were children. Early the next morning Bobby tries to engage a withdrawn DJ into a conversation about the fishing trips they shared in the past. As Bobby reminisces, he and DJ row past a dilapidated castle that captures DJ's interest and sparks a memory. DJ says that he used to dream about that castle, and is delighted to see that it is real. Bobby convinces DJ to explore the castle and rows toward it. DJ goes inside and is suddenly flooded with positive memories.

The next day an animated DJ wakes Bobby up early to go fishing in drenching rain. As they row out, DJ tells Bobby that although he did not want to go fishing, he is so glad he did. DJ says he is finding a sense of purpose. Bobby is astonished as he listens to his brother. "You know what it really is Bobby?" DJ, says, "It's the memories. They're from before. They're so sweet. It's like I go up here and all that sickness never happened here. I can be normal. It's magic," DJ finishes with a broad smile.

As I watched that scene, I fully understood what DJ was trying to communicate. I knew that feeling. I had felt that joy before my abuse, before I had to deal with daily humiliation. Before the beatings that caused my Complex PTSD. Eye Movement Desensitization and Reprocessing (EMDR) is a treatment that helped me to remember happy memories. It was created by psychologist Francine Shapiro, who in 1987 made an observation that by moving her eyes from side to side, she reduced the number of negative thoughts and memories she had previously experienced. She studied her findings while working with initially seventy patients. Dr. Shapiro noticed that EMDR helped guide trauma survivors through their unprocessed memories of trauma by helping them make connections to memories long forgotten by tapping into to the unconscious where many memories, good and bad hide. I was so used to remembering my many horrible memories that I'd blocked out the good ones. Trauma survivors should only seek EMDR therapy from therapists specifically trained and certified to perform

EMDR. It requires the use of alternating sounds or lights to allow trauma survivors to process memories of past trauma. Through EMDR, I could retrieve the wonderful memories of my childhood before we moved to Philadelphia. That was a time in my life that was filled with awe and wonder. Just like DJ said, it was magic.

My first happy memory was crawling on the floor of our apartment in Newark. As I looked up everything seemed so big. We lived in apartment 3D in a tenement building on 232 East Prince Street. I vaguely recall looking up at several tall things. I wasn't quite sure what those tall things were. I was a happy child back then. I don't remember how old I was then. I had my family around me. Our apartment appeared enormous to me at that time. I lived with my mother, my brother Carl who was two years younger than me, my sister Jane who was one year younger than me and my older brother Tony who was three years older than me. When my mother brought my youngest brother Sam home from the hospital that made five of us. I was a big brother once again.

My father did not live with us. I have two memories of him as a child. One was when he stopped by to see us while we were playing outside during a bright summer day. I remember hearing the melodious chimes of an ice cream truck. It was a sound that brought joy to the hearts of children everywhere. It was our hope that someone, anyone would by us an icy treat. On this day, my dad came to the rescue. He bought us, and some of our friends, popsicles. I was happy to see him and I appreciated the popsicles on that hot day. However, he left as quickly as he'd arrived. My last childhood memory of my father was when he had me and my sister Jane over to his apartment. He didn't have much money and had to redeem some soda bottles to buy us a spaghetti dinner. Later that night I wondered who the woman was in the bed with me, Jane and Daddy. She wasn't my mother. I don't think I met her again after that.

My maternal grandparents, Robert and Thelma Hall, along with their teenage sons, Robert, we called him Uncle Robbie, and Moses, we called him Uncle Mosie, lived on the sixth floor of the same building we lived in. My grandfather was a shoe cobbler. He worked hard to support his family. I am reminded of my grandfather whenever I see wingtip shoes. He always wore a shiny pair. I smile when I see a roll top desk because he used to write furiously at his. My grandmother always had a smile for me. My favorite memory of her came after she received a note from my first-grade teacher that stated I had not completed the previous night's reading assignment. She looked at me sternly after reading the note and made me sit in front of her to read while she crocheted. I loved my grandmother and carefully read aloud my missed assignment. What I should tell you is that my grandparents were both deaf and could not read lips. I knew this at that time. It wasn't until much later did I realize that she had no way of knowing if I read my assignment. I did. She told me to do so and I was obedient. My aunt Roberthia, we called her 'Berta never Aunt 'Berta, was like our big sister. She had two sons, our favorite cousins Troy and Marc. They lived in the Spruce Street tenements. I was quite happy with my life at that time.

Early in my childhood, I was considered smart by my uncles Robbie and Mosie. One evening at a family get together my uncles were tickled by the fact at five years old I could spell Mississippi. I have fond memories of graham cracker and milk snacks in kindergarten at Morton Street School. We would take comforting naps in the afternoon. I always enjoyed school. My favorite teacher was Dr. George Cureton, who taught first grade. He was noted for his Action Reading techniques and won a National Teacher award of the year in 1969. He told the children in his class that he was their second father. He spent a lot of time with me and became a father figure to me. I remember his gentle caring spirit. I felt special around him. He even picked me and a few other students from his class to help demonstrate his Action Reading techniques on a PBS television show.

My two best friends in the first grade were Dexter and Robert. They were like brothers to me. I would spend a lot of time before and after school in their apartments. They also lived in tenement buildings. I have fond memories of being warmly greeted by their mothers who would treat me like their son. It was not uncommon for me to arrive at their homes, close to meal time and find a place at the table for me. I often went to their apartments because at that time my mother didn't have enough food for us at home. Despite that, this was one of the happiest times in my life.

One of my fondest memories was going over to Robert's apartment before school. His mother greeted me with a glowing smile as she escorted me to the kitchen. The delicious smell of freshly made pancakes enveloped me, as the sun streamed through the blinds of the kitchen window. I had to shield by eyes from the bright light as I was escorted to my plate of hotcakes. It was so warm and inviting. What a way to start a day, warmth from their love and delicious food.

One of the other happier times in my life was in the summer of 1967. As I was playing with my friends in front of our building we saw a large group of older kids yelling and walking down the street together. When they returned, they threw bags in the air. Suddenly candy rained down on us. It was like Halloween in July. They left and returned in wave after wave and showered us with candy. We were ecstatic. At the end, however, we became dismayed when they started throwing cigarettes and cigars in the air. Our party was over. When I went back to school in the fall, I noticed that our favorite candy store was boarded up. It never reopened. It wasn't until later, that I learned about the Civil Rights protest and the many urban riots. I then realized that we were in the midst of the riots in Newark. Riots that took Newark decades to recover from.

Things became somewhat darker after that summer. I remember hearing the adults talk about maniacs, who would throw people off the roof off our thirteen-story building. The adults would talk about how things were different, somehow more dangerous. They talked about drugs. and about using paddles with nails to "fight the maniacs." They were afraid. I didn't quite understand why. I never saw these maniacs. I did, however, remember feeling quite afraid one night. I overheard my mother tell my aunt that my uncle Mosie was "all cut up." They then rushed from the apartment with a blanket. I had in my mind an image of my uncle cut up in small bloody cubes and they would bring him back on the blanket. Later that night my uncle walked in very much intact with a bandage on his arm.

Despite all the tension in the air, I felt free. I was quite a walker and I walked everywhere. Even though the adults were worried, I was not. Perhaps I was too young to understand the danger. My grandparents did and they wanted me at home before it was dark outside. Although I loved my siblings, I wanted to be with my friends. I was a free spirit, free to wonder about and I loved it. I would visit my aunt, my cousins, and my friends. I have never felt as free as I did then. I was so full of love. There was no doubt that this was the happiest time of my childhood. But that was about to all change.

HURT BURT

My mother and her friend Gene came to visit us in the summer of 1968. We would later call Gene our stepfather even though my mother was separated and still married to my biological father. I never knew why my mother left us with our grandparents. I did know that my grandparents loved us dearly and took good care of us. My mother would return a couple of times with Gene. He seemed like a nice guy, but we resented him because he was not our father. One weekend when my mother came to visit, she told us she would be taking us with her back to Philadelphia. I was devastated. I was being ripped from my family and my dear friends, Robert and Dexter. While I knew in my heart, I would see my family again, I quickly realized I would never see Robert and Dexter again. We wrote letters to each other, but after a few letters we stopped writing.

When we left Newark, we were all huddled in the back seat of Gene's purple Ford Galaxy 500. It was amazing that five kids could all fit. My mother sat in the front passenger's seat while Gene drove. The ride to Philadelphia was long. We stopped along the way at a White Castle restaurant. Gene bought each of us a couple of those delicious little cheeseburgers. Those burgers took away some of the sting of our trip.

It was evening by the time we reached 526 East Penn Street. We were all amazed. We had always lived in a tenement building and everyone we knew lived in a tenement building. But this was a row house! As Gene opened the door we rushed in with childish glee. I noticed a flight of steps. This was amazing to me. I'd never seen a flight of steps inside the place I was living in. In the tenement building, the stairs were outside the apartment. The only time I saw stairs inside a house was while I watched *The Patty Duke Show.* Patty and Cathy Lane would walk down the stairs in their home as the theme song played. I thought it was magical. Now we had stairs in our home. We all ran from room to room. We couldn't believe how big the house was.

We used to sleep in the same room, but now all four boys had a room while Jane had her own room. I thought Jane was so lucky. The bedroom I shared with my brothers was huge. We had far more room than we had in Newark. The newness of this experience dulled the sting of separation from all that was familiar to us. This was a new chapter in my life.

Early in our transition to Philadelphia everything went well. Gene seemed to care about us. He would cook delicious meals for us. We felt so special. My mother seemed happy. One evening she constructed several cardboard boxes with small compartments. She said she was practicing for a test to get a job at the post office. She was placing small pieces of paper in each of the compartments. She eventually got the job at the post office at 30th Street Station. Gene had a job at a furniture factory and seemed to enjoy what he did. In those days, the house was filled with joy. I had no idea that joy would soon disappear.

One day Gene came home, quite upset. I overheard him telling my mother that he had lost his job. I never knew why. I also remember my mother trying to get him a job at the post office. I don't remember if he got it, but I do remember that he became increasingly bitter. We once had more than enough to eat, but now there was not enough for a family of seven. We would often scrounge around in the refrigerator or in the cabinets for food. We innocently thought that there was nothing wrong with getting a snack. We were sadly mistaken. We started to see Gene's dark side.

I don't know if his struggles to find work was what annoyed him or the fact that five little kids required a lot of food. Perhaps he felt that he was losing control over his new family and the pressure was too much to bear. We were eating a lot and my mother was working and he wasn't. All I know is there was now an eerie feeling in our home. Gene began to exert his control over us. We had to ask permission if we wanted to eat anything. This was strange to us since we never had to ask to eat before.

I can't say that I truly remember when he first showed us his anger. It was common for him call us together and ask us who ate some item of food. I knew initially we had all eaten some of the food he was asking about. I often wondered why he asked us that question. What was wrong with us eating when we were hungry? Somehow Gene thought that we had no right to be hungry. To make his point abundantly clear, he asked us to stand side by side, shoulder to shoulder. He would ask each of us with thunder in his voice if we had eaten the food. He was a hulking muscular giant to us. We were still little kids at that time. My brother Tony was nine, I was seven, Jane was six, my brother Carl was five and my brother Sam was two. Fearful, none of us would admit to eating anything. Gene, in his flawed logic, decided that since no one would admit to eating the food, he would have to beat all of us. He considered that being fair. In his flawed logic, beating little children for being hungry was the right thing to do. He never thought that perhaps we needed more food and he should reassure us instead of beating us. He never considered that these frightened kids would benefit from a hug. He could have used that incident as a teachable moment. He could have stressed the importance of telling the truth. It could have been a moment we grew closer to him. Instead, the worst possible thing happened.

Gene unplugged an extension cord from an outlet. One by one he demanded that we enter an adjacent room where he beat us with the cord. This happened several times. I was never the first one. That honor went to Tony as Gene would beat us oldest to youngest. I was usually second. Fear engulfed me as I heard my older brother Tony being beaten. The sound of the extension cord as it whistled through the air, the sound it made as it struck Tony's back, buttocks and legs coupled with his screams of pain scared me to my very core.

The wait for my turn was unbearable. Tears streamed from my eyes and my hands trembled as I tried to make sense of the senseless. Why would Gene beat us for eating when we were hungry I wondered? When it was my turn I entered the room. Gene wore a mask of anger. He tightened his grip on the extension cord. This was a surreal experience. Never in my life had anyone showed me so much animosity. My mother was at home at the time. She sat in another room. She never intervened. The whistle of the extension cord was far more frightening when directed at me. Each time I was struck, I screamed in pain as I felt the burning sting of the cord. I would tense up as I waited for the next blow. It seemed to go on forever. Finally, mercifully, it was over. I quickly scurried to another room to join Tony. When it was all over I would look around the room we all sat in. we whimpered as we looked at each other. I saw a look of disbelief on their tear soaked faces of my siblings. I looked at the back of my legs and saw welts and abrasions. The physical scars paled in comparison to the deep wounds beginning to form in my psyche.

That was the beginning of the loss of my childhood innocence. Slowly my free-spirited nature would leave me, replaced by the cancer of shame and guilt. In Newark, I walked the streets with my head up and shoulders thrown back as if I owned the city. I didn't have a care in the world then. One beating rocked that confidence. Despite living in a city with a recent history of civil unrest, I felt safe in Newark. In a short period of time, my world became a scary place as the beatings continued regularly. I walked around now with my head lowered; my back hunched over as I cowered in fear. The world was no longer a safe place.

My siblings and I endured several horrific beatings. We were at Gene's mercy. I felt all alone. No one came to our rescue, not even our mother. There were a few beatings that stood out to me. My third-grade teacher, Mrs. Bauman, wanted to have a small meeting with me and a few of my classmates at John Wister Elementary School. The night before the meeting I was beaten. I would usually go to school and act as if nothing had happened. On this day, I remember slowly walking into a chilly room. I limped to the wooden table where the students were all gathered. I walked methodically, careful not to wince in pain. I did not want to attract any attention. I slowly lowered myself onto a chair. I felt the cold hard wood against the tender welts on my thighs and back through my clothes. I wished the meeting would end quickly so I could leave and suffer in silence.

Another memory was one that occurred right before I received a beating. I did not feel safe eating at the dining room table. I did not feel safe around Gene or my mother. I had a habit of putting food in my pocket and going to my third-floor bedroom to eat it. On this occasion, Gene found that I had cake in my pocket. He had asked me why I put food in my pocket . I thought I could challenge his assumption. I was smart, my uncles told me so. I said that I didn't have food in my pocket, I had cake, that's a dessert. Gene ridiculed me and said I was wrong, cake was food. Then he used a profanity laced tirade to ridicule me even more before he beat me. At that moment, I doubted my own intellect and have done so on many occasions after that.

Finally, the one beating that still echoes in my soul was one I witnessed when I was nine years-old. My brother, I won't identify who because that is not as important. My brother had eaten something and Gene knew he did it. Gene decided he would not beat all of us just my brother. He said. "I'm going to beat you until I'm tired." Those words were scary enough, but what happened next was far more frightening. He tied my poor brother to a bed with a rope from a clothesline. He then proceeded to beat him with an extension cord.

My brother had been wearing a pair of corduroy pants. My brother shrieked in both horror and pain as Gene relentlessly beat him. He beat him so hard that my brother's pants shredded. I remember seeing pieces of it torn away by the extension cord to reveal bloody welts on his legs. My brother was in so much pain that in a burst of adrenaline, he broke out of his restraints and ran out of the room. Gene mercifully did not follow after him. I was frozen in fear and could not believe what I just witnessed. I also felt ashamed that I did not come to my brother's defense. For a few days after the beating he couldn't walk and was bedridden. About a week later, he would limp around the house with a childish smile on his face. He was coping with what happened better than I was. I shoved the memory of that beating into the recesses of my mind. Today, I cannot. To heal I must deal with this and other terrible memories.

There were many more beatings to follow. Each one seemed to wipe away the smile I once had in my soul. Gene wasn't only satisfied with controlling us within the walls of our home. He also wanted to control our lives outside as well. Not only did we have to ask for permission to eat, we had to ask for permission to go outside and play. Part of the joy of childhood is the freedom to play. Even inside the house our laughter seemed to annoy Gene. We were not to be seen or heard.

On many a bright sunny day as we heard our friends gleefully playing outside and many days we could only watch them.

We could only go outside if Gene was in a good mood. As a young child, I had chores to perform. I had no issue with that, what bothered me was my expectation that after finishing my chores, I would be allowed to go outside. That was not always the case. Gene was sadistic. There was no way of knowing with any certainty how to make him happy. If we didn't follow his rules, we faced a beating. If we did follow his rules, we could be ignored, verbally abused for bothering him, or on rare occasions acknowledged in a positive manner. On several occasions, I would sheepishly cower as I approached him to ask if I could go outside. I would tiptoe as I walked towards him. I would try to read his nonverbal signals in hopes that I could predict a positive outcome.

When he was not home and we wanted to go outside, we would ask my mother. If our chores were done, she would allow us to go out to play. My sister had her friends she would play with. My brothers and I enjoyed playing sports. We would play baseball, basketball and football. We chose what game to play based on the sport season. Many a game was interrupted when our sister would tell us that Gene wanted us to come home. I felt both dejected and humiliated as I walked back home. I knew I faced a verbal barrage at minimum, and sometimes a beating. My childhood was a rollercoaster ride of mostly negative emotions.

One way I learned to cope was by drawing. I started drawing because of my love of comic books. I discovered comic books at a young age. Like many kids, I loved watching cartoons. I felt that comic books represented cartoons I could hold in my hands. I guess what fascinated me was their bright colors. I didn't see cartoons on television in color until I was a pre-teen. A color television was a luxury item. Not many families I knew could afford one. We could not. The first comic book I saw was ripped pages from a *Fantastic Four* Marvel comic book I saw on the ground on my way to school. The brilliant colors fascinated me. I'd watched the *Fantastic Four* cartoon on a black and white television and now I had what I thought was the actual cartoon in my hand.

I became intrigued with the artwork in the comic book. I would go to the neighborhood drug store and buy three comic books that had the cover partially cut off for twenty-five cents instead of the regular forty-five cents price. Many lonely days were spent in the bedroom I shared with my brothers, drawing picture after picture. I dreamt of being a comic book artist when I grew up. I even made up a superhero group called the Illusion Brothers. Each of my brothers was a member.

Drawing was such a relief for me. I loved the process of illustrating my favorite superheroes. I admired the artwork of great comic book artists like John Buscema, Neal Adams, Jack Kirby and Murphy Anderson. Whenever I would draw or read my comics, I was transported to a magical world inhabited by super beings who went to fascinating places. I was transported to a world devoid of the pain and suffering I had to endure. My fantasy was that I would pursue a career drawing comic books.

One thing that made me consider another career path was my mother's pursuit of her education. She had dropped out of high school. She lived in rural Georgia and had to help support her family. After we moved to Philadelphia she applied for and was able to receive public assistance to help provide support for us, but she had no desire to stay on welfare. She had bigger aspirations. Despite having to care for five little children, she decided to pursue her GED. After earning it, she told Gene that her welfare case manager wanted her to apply for menial jobs. She decided instead to pursue a career in nursing. As I looked through her nursing textbooks I developed an interest in medicine.

It didn't take long before Gene tried to thwart her efforts. My mother would spend long hours at school. Gene expected her to cook dinner every day while he waited. Many times, he didn't even eat what she made. Several nights he would start to eat, then fall asleep with half eaten food on his plate. He then started to accuse my mother of having an affair because she was spending so much time studying. This was strange because it was common for women to call our home asking for Gene. Once my mother had a meeting with her classmates and arrived home late. Gene became irate when she came home. He started to yell at her and to beat her. I was terrified. I was about nine years old and terribly afraid of him. I was frozen. Just like when my brother was beaten while being tied down. I couldn't move.

In the middle of beating my mother Gene picked up the telephone and struck her on the head with it several times. My mother shrieked in pain. I heard the disconcerting chime of the bell inside the phone as he struck her on the head with it. My heart sank. I was trembling as I stood there watching. I hoped that he would stop and eventually he did. After he was finished assaulting her, he got dressed and left the house, slamming the door on his way out. My siblings and I tried to comfort my mother who was now quietly sobbing. Her face was contorted and covered with cuts and bruises. Her eyes were swollen shut. I looked at the sea green telephone. Those Bell telephones were sturdy. Gene had struck my mother so hard that the base of the phone cracked. My mother had to miss a few days of school. When she finally left the house, she wore dark sunglasses with big lenses. We never talked about that incident. I wish I could say that was the only time Gene hit my mother, it wasn't. There were other times. That particular time was the most brutal.

What impressed me about that period of my life was how my mother persisted in pursuing her education. I admired her courage. She was able to take care of us to the best of her ability and cope with an unsupportive, jealous and abusive paramour and still graduate from nursing school. When she graduated, I thought, if she could do it so could I. I decided to pursue a career in medicine. My mother gave me the confidence to believe that despite hardship and struggle, I could do it. Her triumph gave me hope.

I spent a great deal of my life in nearly constant state of fear. Between the ages of six to about ten beatings were a regular occurrence. This set the stage for an atmosphere of perpetual fear at home. I always had a sense of uneasiness. I would isolate myself in my third-floor bedroom away from Gene, my mother, and even my siblings. Whenever I was around Gene, I carefully analyzed his nonverbal cues. I could relax when he would laugh although I had to be alert for sudden changes in his mood. Little things like, if we didn't do our chores the way wanted us to, or if dinner was not prepared to his liking, would send him into a rage. The bellow of his voice was frightening to me.

I was most relaxed when he would take a bath as he prepared to go on a date with one of his many women. We would hear Gene playing Lou Rawls' *It Was a Very Good Year* on his record players, as he whistled while he dressed. Gene prided himself on the many flashy suits he owned. We on the other hand wore hand-me-downs. I would bag groceries at an Acme supermarket to make enough money to buy clothes from the Thrift store on Germantown Avenue. Gene on the other hand was a sharp dresser. I would listen in careful anticipation as he prepared to go out. I knew once he left, I could relax and enjoy being a child for a little while.

When Gene was gone, a brightness permeated throughout the house. I would laugh and joke with my siblings. We would watch television together. Those would be the times we would spend time showing our mother love. As Gene would often spend nights away, we would get a chance to sleep in our mother's bed. Those were some of the most restful sleeps we would have. My mother would share her dreams with us. She didn't learn to drive until she was nearly thirty, but she would tell us that when she got her driver's license she would take us to the Philadelphia Zoo or the Franklin Institute. I smiled so wide when she first told us this. My mother seemed happiest when Gene was away. We were very different when he wasn't there. We were a family. When Gene was around we were all scattered, hiding, and trembling in fear.

The slam of the front door when Gene returned home would shatter our sense of peace and harmony. He would slam it with such force that the house shook. I could hear his footsteps on the wooden floors. Often there would be an eerie silence after a few steps. On several occasions that would be followed by a piercing whistle. He would often whistle as a signal to call us downstairs. This whistle was always a harbinger of something horrible, a profanity laced verbal barrage or possibly a beating. The slam of that front door always engendered fear.

To me that fear was a lot more than an emotional state, it was something that latched onto my soul. It was the atmosphere I existed in when I was at home. It threatened to take my very breath away. It certainly usurped any remnants of happiness I felt at that time. When I was older I tried to convince myself that the fear was gone, but all it took was the slam of a door, a loud voice or a noisy crowd for me to feel that fear again. The fear wasn't just at home, it was everywhere because it was inside of me.

Holidays were also a source of stress for us. When we arrived in Philadelphia, we expected small birthday gifts. My favorite gift for one of my birthdays was two books. One was *Seven With One Blow*. It was a magical tale about a tailor who could kill seven flies with one stroke of his belt. The other was *Caps For Sale*, about a man who sold a lot of hats. I was so surprised to receive those books and I read them several times because I was a voracious reader. Sometimes at Christmas we would each receive several gifts. There was many a Christmas eve when we couldn't go to sleep. We were too excited thinking about the gifts we would receive. The first one who woke up Christmas day would wake the others and we would all run downstairs. Christmas and Thanksgiving were holidays when we ate well. Those were the only times in the year when we ate until we were full.

Things began to change by the time I was in the fifth grade. There were no birthday gifts. There were many Christmases where we received no gifts. Our first Christmas without gifts the tree was not even lit. Even though there were no gifts, I didn't find it strange because in the past the tree was bare until Christmas morning, but there were always Christmas lights. My siblings and I had trouble sleeping Christmas eve, which was normal. When we ran downstairs we found the unlit Christmas tree with no gifts beneath it. We were surprised, shocked and disappointed. The hurt I felt was far more painful than any beating.

The following Christmas, we didn't even have a tree. Christmas morning, we tiptoed down the stairs hoping against hope that we would have at least one gift. I stood midway on the stairs and looked down. There was still no tree and no gifts. I walked back up to my bedroom and tried go to sleep. I could hear the laughter of the kids in the neighborhood riding bicycles or playing with the toys they received. I think that the saddest thing that we had to endure was the silence. There was no explanation, or comfort from my mother or Gene. We couldn't comfort each other since we were all suffering. As I write this I think about the lyrics from *The Little Boy That Santa Claus Forgot*. It echoes the sadness I felt on Christmas when there was nothing under the tree.

For years, I would become depressed as my birthday approached because it was such a reminder of painful childhood memories of times when I didn't receive a gift. Christmas was even worse. When I saw stores putting up Christmas decorations my heart sank. I would be barraged with Christmas carols. The Sunday paper would be stuffed with a huge toys section so kids could make up their list. It is funny how all these things can be traumatizing to a child who knows that there will be no gifts for him. By the time I returned to school after not receiving a present I had cried my last tears. This was the beginning of me wearing the mask that would cover my pain. During recess, as I played with my friends, someone asked what everyone got for Christmas. I felt frozen, not from the frosty air, but from the question. The other kids chimed in but I had no reply. I suddenly no longer felt like I was okay. I think I became aware of how different I was from my peers. I began to feel less than them. I wondered if my parents loved me as much as their parents loved them.

I would be remiss if I characterized my childhood as an entirely negative experience. There were a few things that we enjoyed doing. One thing we enjoyed was expressing our hatred for Gene. Of course, we only did this when he was not at home. The other thing was fantasizing about our biological father. To a child, Philadelphia was light years away from Newark. We thought our father didn't know where we were because if he did, he would beat up Gene and take us back to Newark. Another highlight of our childhood was the vacations we spent in Newark staying with Aunt 'Berta, Uncle Steve and our favorite cousins, the only cousins we knew, Troy and Marc.

Aunt Berta and Uncle Steve showed us love. They were genuinely interested in us. I felt I was transported back to the time we lived in Newark. Newark Burt would resurface and I would be happy and carefree. Berta and Steve allowed us to be kids. They never tried to micromanage our lives like Gene. We would go out and play all day with Troy and Marc. We would return and they would have delicious meals for us. They enjoyed our company and we enjoyed theirs. We were a well-behaved lot, so discipline was hardly necessary, but when it was needed, Uncle Steve sat us down and had a compassionate conversation with us. We were never beaten or scolded.

While in Newark, we would visit my maternal grandparents who always had a warm smile for us. My mother had two brothers, but we never visited them. They had children who we never knew. As much as we fantasized about our father while we were in Philadelphia, we never thought about him while we were in Newark. He also never seemed to know we were in Newark. At least that was what I thought since he never stopped by to see us.

There was once an urgent call Berta made to my mother when I was about fourteen or fifteen. My father had suffered a stroke and was hospitalized in Newark. He reached out to my aunt in the hope she would speak to my mother. He wanted to see us. My mother asked us if we wanted to see our father. We did. We took the train to Newark because I guess Gene didn't want to drive to

Newark. Berta and Steve took us to the hospital. I remember seeing him lying in the bed, he looked frail, like a shell of a man. His eyes were filled with anguish and tears streamed down his face. He was not able to talk or move his arms. He had dried mucous in his moustache. I carefully removed it with a tissue. He lay there motionless as more tears fell from his eyes. We each told him we loved him. He was no longer the hulking man I once knew. The man who used to call me "champ" looked defeated. It was so sad seeing him like this. That day the dream of him rescuing us died. He was clearly no match for Gene.

As much as we enjoyed our trips to Newark, it was so painful leaving. We would hug 'Berta and Uncle Steve for a long time, but we would each hug Troy and Marc for what seemed an eternity. I felt like my heart was being ripped to shreds when I had to leave them. Their tears told me they felt the same way. I sobbed as I looked at Troy and Marc waving to us as we drove away. A part of me always stayed behind. The part of me that was Newark Burt. That part was always there for me when I returned. We all cried all the way home to Philadelphia. I could feel myself transformed from the fiercely independent child I was in Newark to the frightened trembling child I was in Philadelphia as soon I entered the car.

Before my mother finished nursing school, we received public assistance. She would receive a food voucher and eventually food stamps once a month. At the first of the month Gene would take my mother shopping. She would return with several bags of groceries. We would have delicious meals during the first few weeks of the month. By the end of the month there were only leftovers. My mother would take the bone from the ham she'd bought in the beginning of the month and cook it with dry beans such as lima beans and black-eyed beans. Although lima beans and black-eyed beans are delicious, I no longer eat them because I associate them with the poverty of my youth.

During the times when we had plenty to eat Gene would make his infamous banana pudding. It was a delicious recipe he made that included fresh bananas, vanilla wafers and condensed milk. He enjoyed making it and we enjoyed when he made because he was always in a good mood when he prepared it. He topped it with a meringue that was slightly toasted on the top. We all giggled as it baked. Its wonderful aroma filled the entire house. He would serve us generous portions.

As good as this confection was, it also was a source of pain. Inevitably, one of my siblings would sneak another serving at night. Gene would ask who did it. No one would confess, so we all would receive a beating. This wonderful desert was now a source of pain for me. I stopped eating it.   Gene would excuse me from the beatings since he knew I did not like it. I did like it, but eating it was not worth the pain associated with it. Gene's mind functioned quite simply. I could have still eaten it secretly and got away with it because he thought I didn't like it. There was no way I could be so treacherous. I could not place my siblings in such jeopardy, knowing I would be excused from a beating and they were not. I had received more than my share of beatings for things I didn't do. I did not want to do that to them. If Gene ever found out I had deceived him, the beating he would have given me would been worse than the one my brother got when he was tied to the bed.

At this point, I started to withdraw from my family. I also would not accept anything from Gene when he was in a good mood because he would use any positive feelings against you. That point was hammered home one Christmas. Gene asked us every year to write a list of things we wanted. As small children, we would take pleasure in making our list. We would look at the toy section in the Sunday paper and write our list. We would then discuss what we had written, then give the lists to Gene. He would take them but he would buy whatever he wanted. Often what he bought us was not on any of our lists.

One Christmas, I did get what I wanted. I was eleven years old. I asked for a typewriter and I got it. I remember being filled with a strange emotion at that time. It was beyond happiness, it was joy. It overwhelmed me. It was so foreign to me I became scared. I thought I was going to die. I, Hurt Burt, got what I wanted. Me, the child filled with shame and low self-esteem finally got what he wanted. I felt I was at the zenith of my life. My life had to be over. It wasn't. That moment became etched in my mind as I tapped into it several times afterward. It was so hard to accept anything positive when you swim in the sea of despair.

I apologize for that digression. One Christmas, when I was fifteen, I told Gene, I didn't want anything. He had asked my siblings to make their lists, which they did. I didn't because I knew at this point that he would buy us whatever he wanted. I was also still scarred by the Christmases where there were no gifts as well the chronic emotional abuse. I didn't want to be hurt again. Gene kept asking me if I wanted anything and I kept saying no. On Christmas day after everyone received their gifts, he looked at me and said, "Burt, I really feel bad that you didn't get anything." He then reached in his wallet and gave me a twenty-dollar bill, which was a lot of money to me. He then looked at me with tears streaming from his eyes and said, "Merry Christmas." I was shocked. I didn't know what to do. He had never shown me this level of vulnerability or affection.

Later that day, Gene was playing his music and getting ready to go out. He called me down from my bedroom and said, "Listen, I'm going to have to borrow that twenty dollars I gave you. I'll give it back to you when I get paid on Friday." I gave it back to him. He finished dressing and went out and I have not seen that twenty dollars since. That moment cemented in my mind that I could never trust Gene.

As a young child, I absolutely adored my mother. It was more of an innate love than one based on any specific memories. I have a few memories of my mother when I lived in Newark. I remember I received more love and affection from the mothers of my friends Dexter and Robert than I did from my own mother. She took care of us as kids, but I don't recall any particularly tender moments. Yet I had a great deal of affection for her all the same. When I was in elementary school I earned a dollar from cleaning a neighbor's basement. I went to Woolworth's, looking for a Christmas gift for my mother. I wanted to get her something nice. I felt she deserved it because she was my mom. I thought she was so smart. I would ask her questions and she always had an answer. She was so bright. I began to see her brightness dim when Gene would abuse her. My mother would spend a lot of time in bed when Gene was not at home. I'm sure my mother was suffering from some form of depression back then.

My love for my mother began to fade when I was in the tenth grade. I was involved in Junior Achievement. Our project was to make a pillow out of t-shirts that we stuffed and then used iron-on letters to personalize. I was a shy child and Junior Achievement helped me come out of my shell. I went to Central High School, at that time it was a boys-only academic public high school. One of my classmates, Benjamin, was in the program with me. There were also kids, including girls, from other high schools there. It was my one opportunity to interact with girls, some of whom were quite cute.

I was excited about our project. I got up one morning to meet up with my teammates to start assembling our t-shirt pillows. As I poured a glass of milk I told my mother about my plans for the day. I told her about the project several days earlier and she'd said I could go. When I finished drinking my milk, she looked at me and said, "You need to do your chores first." I promised her that I would finish my chores when I got back. She said, "Gene wants you to do your chores, you can't go." I was hurt because she knew I always did my chores and that the project was important to me. What hurt me the most was that she would not advocate for me.

I didn't go that day. I completed my chores as I was instructed to do. When I finished, it was too late to meet my friends. I felt ashamed and humiliated. I tried to avoid Benjamin at school the following week. I was too embarrassed to tell him that I was not allowed to go. When I finally met, him face to face, I gave him some lame excuse. I never went back to Junior Achievement. I decided not to become involved with any extracurricular activities. I was fearful that I would not be able to continue and have to make up stupid excuses as to why I couldn't be there. This I believed cost me dear relationships with classmates in high school when many of them were beginning to exert their independence. Not me. I was a prisoner in my own home. I was a slave to shame and wallowed in a well of low self-esteem.

Another event that significantly affected me was when my oldest brother Tony was kicked out of the house. When he was about sixteen, he started hanging out with the wrong crowd and would stay out all night. He started drinking alcohol and perhaps even smoked marijuana. One day he was so drunk he passed out and vomited all over the couch in the living room. Gene told him to stop hanging out with his friends. Gene would even assault him, but Tony wouldn't listen. One day Gene gave him an ultimatum. He told Tony that if he stayed out one more night he would kick him out of the house. Tony still stayed out and Gene did indeed kick him out. I overheard the conversation between Gene and my mother. He said he had to kick Tony out to set an example for us. Gene felt that if he allowed Tony to continue this behavior, the rest of us would follow suit. So, he kicked Tony out to teach him a lesson. That single move sent my brother on a downward spiral that impacts his life even today.

Gene told us that since he kicked Tony out we were not allowed to let him in or to help him in any way. I felt so afraid for Tony. I knew he had nowhere to go. He needed help. He would knock on the kitchen window after Gene left and ask for something to eat. I wanted to help him but I was afraid. I didn't want Gene to kick me out too. I knew Tony was hungry. I felt like a coward because I was paralyzed by fear, my sister Jane however, did not feel as I did. She allowed Tony to come in and wash up. She fed him. She was courageous, I was not. She risked her own safety. I would beat myself up emotionally for my inability to move beyond my fear to help my brother.

Tony dislocated his shoulder while he was out on his own. Gene allowed him to come back home while his arm healed. Tony started drinking alcohol again and was kicked out again. He would often break into the house when we were in school. He would steal my clothes since we wore the same size. I was mad at first, but I eventually understood that he needed them more than I did. I fantasized that he would overcome this period of his life. I envisioned that there would be a time when he would get an apartment and invite me over and give me brotherly advice. I imagined he would tell me that he was alright. That day never came. I dealt with his life situation in the only way I knew how. I pretended that he didn't exist. I blamed him initially, wondering why couldn't he just stop drinking? I then realized that he was a child. He needed what we'd never gotten from Gene or our mother. He needed compassion. He needed help. I doubled down on my pursuit to be the perfect child. I didn't want to be kicked out for not following the rules no matter how insane those rules were.

Jane showed me courage in another way. When she turned eighteen she moved out of the house. She didn't want to live under Gene's tyranny. She was also angry at my mother for allowing Gene to abuse us. When she left, we were forbidden to speak to her. I was proud that she had the courage to seek her own serenity. She has been and continues to be courageous.

What forever fractured my relationship with my mother was when she asked me to leave the house in December of 1981. I returned home from school a year earlier in 1979 after flunking out of my first semester at Temple University. I had received educational grants and financial aid which paid for my tuition and housing but not for meals. I had to work at Gino's, a fast food restaurant to pay for my meals. My plan was that I would work the night shift and go to school during the day. I was also involved in a relationship at that time.

To support myself and maintain a social life, I would work long hours. I was dating one of my co-workers and I would take the last bus home with her to make sure she got there safely. I would sleep on the living room sofa at her house until early the next morning I would then take the first bus in the morning to my dorm to sleep. This would cause me to over sleep. I would wake up late and miss classes. During finals week of the fall semester of 1979, I was running around Temple University campus trying to find out where my finals were being held. Since I didn't go to class, I didn't know where to go. Even if I had known, I would not have done well because I hadn't studied. When I got my grades, I had failed all my classes except chemistry lab. The graduate student running the class generously gave me a C. I didn't deserve it.

I scheduled a meeting with my academic advisor at Temple University and asked if I could be given another chance. She suggested that I attend a community college instead so I enrolled at the Community College of Philadelphia. My relationship had ended, the only thing I had to focus on was school. I had to atone for the mistake I made at Temple University. I did well at Community College of Philadelphia, and made the honor roll my first year. It was important to me to get good grades since I wanted to go to medical school. I thought everything was going well until that faithful morning. My mother kicked me out the house, I suppose, for getting up early to study for my organic chemistry class. I couldn't face the truth was that neither she nor Gene was supportive of me.

Organic chemistry was difficult for me and I was determined to do well. I woke up before Gene, which seemed to disturb him. He and my mother had a whispered conversation in their bedroom. I was getting dressed in the back room on the second floor. My mother came in and said words that rocked my foundation. "Gene says you have to move out." I was in a state of disbelief. I was being kicked out for getting up before Gene. This made no sense to me. Perhaps Gene was too scared to ask me to leave because he was afraid of me.

I had been lifting weights and I was quite muscular at that time. Maybe he thought that I would beat him up if he told me to leave. I don't know. I had considered myself a good kid. In my neighborhood any parent would have been glad to have me as their son. I did well in school, that one semester at Temple University aside. I had a part-time job and contributed to the family. I was not on drugs, never suspended from school and never arrested. In most families, that was to be expected, but in my family, my neighborhood, I was a unicorn, a rare child indeed. I thought I'd done everything to please them, but apparently, I had not.

I pleaded with my mother but she gave me only a blank stare. Her eyes were without compassion. I was devastated. How could the mother I loved so much, do this to me? It was something I expected from Gene. It hurt me deeply hearing her say those worlds. To say I felt like the rug was pulled from under me would be an understatement. I felt like my heart was being ripped out my chest bit by bit with an ice pick. The stabs of this deep betrayal were so painful. My mother, my inspiration for my decision to seek a career in medicine, had betrayed me.

A few days later in the evening I had a conversation with Gene on the front porch of our home. I wanted to negotiate a truce. I told him about my future plans. I would complete my Associates degree in the next year and then contribute financially in a more substantial way. What he said seemed to me like utter nonsense. He said, "I don't want you to leave, your mother does." I couldn't accept that. I was sure he was lying, but at least he didn't ask me to leave. I thought I was out of danger until a few days later my mother said to me, "Gene says you got to leave today."

In a daze, I packed up my clothing and about forty comic books, which fit into a small box. My comics were my prized possession. At that time, the only other children in the house were my two youngest brothers and my youngest sister, Kiana. She was the lovechild of Gene and my mother. She was eleven years younger than me. She had not endured the hardships we'd endured. When she was born, my mother had finished nursing school and our family was in a better financial position.

When I left home, there was no one to wish me well. I called my dear friend Courtland Kanzinger. Court was the first angel God placed in my life. We met at the YMCA on Greene Street in the

Germantown section of Philadelphia where we both worked out. One day we just started talking and I was surprised by how well we got along. We had so many differences that should make it difficult for us to be friends. Those differences were not significant in the end. He was a middle-aged Christian Caucasian man, twenty-seven years older than me. He grew up in the Maine Line, a wealthy suburban section outside of Philadelphia. He never married and did not have any children. He was close to his loving family and I had the pleasure to meet some of them. His father was a pastor and he was raised in a Christian home.

I can only credit God's providence to explain how I had the opportunity to meet Courtland F. Kanzinger. He preferred to be called Court. He entered my life when I craved a father figure. He exceeded my expectations. He would take me out to dinner and to museums. What I loved the most about Court was how he expanded my world view. Before Court, all I knew was my immediate surroundings. I would catch a glimpse of how the rich and famous lived on television. I knew that it would be next to impossible for me to live the way they did. Often after dinner, we would drive around the suburbs. I was amazed by the sheer numbers and sizes of the houses outside of Philadelphia.

I started thinking differently about my future, that I could have a life different than what I was living. I imagined a brighter future. The greatest gift God has given me is allowing me to meet Court. Court never asked for anything from me other than my friendship. He showed me kindness at a time in my life when I needed it the most. He has since gone on to be with the Lord, but I will never forget him. I thank God for Courtland F. Kanzinger. After I left my childhood home, Court allowed me to stay with him for a few days. He lived in Upper Darby which wasn't convenient for me for school and work. I called Jane and she let me stay in her one bedroom apartment she shared with her boyfriend. It was in Germantown, which made it easier for me to get to school and work.

That was a surreal period in my life. At least I had a way of supporting myself. I was a research assistant at the department of Anesthesia at Temple University Hospital. The ironic thing was that my mother worked as a nurse in the recovery room at the same hospital. The recovery room provided medical support for patients after they had surgery. It was the anesthesiologist who would escort the post-operative patients to the recovery room. The department of Anesthesiology was about fifty feet away, which meant I had to walk by the recovery room at least three to four times a week.

One day while walking down the corridor that lead to the recovery room I felt a dark cold pain as I walked by. I could not turn my head and look at the door leading into the recovery room because I knew my mother was there interacting with her peers as if nothing had happened, as if she had not ripped a hole in my soul. This pain quickly began to manifest as anger but I refused to allow it to destroy me. I would continue in school. I was determined to do well, which I did. I viewed what had happened to me as Gene and my mother's way of derailing my dreams. Instead it gave me a steely resolve. I also vowed to never ask them if I could return. I never wanted to. I never trusted Gene, I knew I could not trust my mother.

I hated Gene and my mother for what they had done to me. Since I felt that they didn't want me to be successful I was more determined than ever to succeed. I focused on the goal to be the best student I could be. I appreciated the opportunity to live with my sister. I was resolved not to be a burden to her. I worked as a chemistry tutor at Community College in addition to the job at Temple University Hospital. I shared my earnings with Jane.

Jane did her best to make me feel comfortable. I slept on the sofa in her living room. When I wasn't studying, I spent a great deal of time wallowing in self-pity. I felt so empty inside but I would not allow myself to experience the full depth of my pain. I did, however allow it to touch the tender emotional periphery of my heart. My first love, my mother, had betrayed me. I was totally blindsided, didn't see it coming. I vowed to never let anyone get that close to me. I was not interested in dating at that time. All I wanted to do was attend classes, study, work and sleep.

While working as a tutor I met my first wife, Sharon. She was quiet and rarely asked any questions. I thought it was because she didn't understand what I was trying to teach. That was not the case, since she was getting an A in her chemistry class. I wasn't sure why she was in my tutoring class. She had a delicate smile and piercing eyes. She faithfully attended all my tutoring sessions. I worked as a tutor for about a year and was offered a job as a chemistry lab assistant. The job paid more so I jumped at the opportunity. Shortly after I started working there, Sharon was hired.

A co-worker suggested that I ask her out, which I did. I remember feeling awkward around her. I didn't trust her. I felt she would hurt me like my mother had. Over time I became fond of her. She had a loving family. I was occasionally invited to her family home over for Sunday dinners. She lived with her parents, her older sister, and younger brother. Her mother greeted me warmly, just like the mothers of my friends back in Newark.

During the first dinners; I was extremely polite. I wanted more than one serving of food, but modesty prevented me from asking. Her mother insisted that I eat more each time I ate with them. I would decline her offer initially but the food was delicious so eventually I decided to have another helping. I was never used to having more than one serving of food at any meal except for Thanksgiving and Christmas. Sharon's sister and brother laughed at me when they recounted how I much food I ate that day years later. They couldn't believe how I wolfed down the food as if I had never eaten before. Sharon's family was so warm and inviting. They were nothing like my family. I really enjoyed being around them.

This new relationship was unsettling for me in the beginning. I kept waiting for Sharon to become bored with me. She never did.

On one occasion, she said a few words that were disturbing to me. She looked me in the eyes and she said, "I love you." At the age of nineteen, I had never heard those words. My deaf grandparents would use sign language to say they loved me, but no one had ever said it to me. My mother never did, 'Berta and Uncle Steve never did, and certainly Gene never did. Here was this beautiful 19-year-old woman, saying these words to me. I was startled for a second, then I said, "Why did you say that?" She looked shocked. I don't think she was expecting that response. I had not been used to anyone saying anything as wonderful as those three words. I didn't feel worthy of them. I did not feel lovable. I had a hard time accepting the truth of her words. I became more attached to her and fell in love with her. I eventually spent more and more time with her family and less time at Jane's apartment.

While living with Jane, she would share with me letters she received from our father. He was in failing health. He'd been plagued by alcoholism and had never taken care of himself. He had high blood pressure and had several strokes. His handwriting had deteriorated into a scrawl that was at times illegible. He wanted his children to visit him and would send a few dollars in his letters.

Since Jane and I were cast out from the family, we had very little contact with my siblings who still lived at home. We also had no idea where Tony was. We wanted to see our father and decided to go. We would have liked to ask the others if they wanted to go with us but that was not an option open to us.

Neither one of us had seen our father since we visited after his first stroke several years ago. Since then he'd had several strokes. He now lived in a skilled nursing facility nestled within tenement buildings. His complex was designed for senior citizens, which was odd since our father was in his early forties. When we got off the train in Newark, we took a cab ride to his apartment. It was surrounded by tenement buildings in a dilapidated section of Newark. As we got out of the cab, I was amazed at the enormity of the tenements that dwarfed my father's complex. That section of the city had not fared well during the Newark riots. Several of the windows were broken and the few bare trees were covered in trash. I felt bad that my father had to live in an area with huge abandoned buildings. I thought we were the only people there until I heard a woman yelling out from the upper floors of the adjacent tenement building. She was talking to a woman who was walking toward the entrance. The buildings weren't abandoned, they were just not well maintained.

We had to be buzzed into his apartment. He slowly opened the door. As he opened the door I noticed that his eyes were full of sadness and despair. He looked even more frail than he had a few years ago. He had to walk with a cane and his right arm had atrophied. It was much smaller than his left arm. His speech was hard to understand and his voice was low and he stuttered. He didn't have much in his apartment. I noticed was that he had a rowing exercise machine. I wondered what value that machine was to him now. My father said people from his church were shopping for food for him. Jane looked in his kitchen cabinets and saw that he had a few can of vegetables. There wasn't much more in the refrigerator. Jane and I were shocked to see him like this. We looked at each other and shook our heads. I felt sad because I knew we only had enough money to get back to Philadelphia. We had no money to give him.

Despite the fact he didn't have much, my father felt the need to give us something, I tried to tell him no, but he insisted that I take something. He gave me his driver's license. He wanted me to renew it for him before it expired. I thought that was strange. I tried to tell him that he would have to be the one to renew it. I guess he thought that he was transferring his license to me since we both had the same name. He was insistent. It was pointless for me to debate the issue with him, so I took the license. I had very few memories of my father before that day, but of the ones I had I remembered him as a vibrant man. He was no longer that man.

After returning to Philadelphia, I focused on my education. I shared my dream of pursuing a career in medicine with Sharon and she was supportive. She wasn't exactly sure what career she was interested in so I encouraged her to consider what she wanted to do. Just like me, she was an honor student. Although it was painful to do, I shared with her the painful memories of my childhood. She listened attentively. We began to spend a lot of time together. We were committed to each other and we decided to get married in the summer of 1982. We didn't have much money. We had a civil ceremony with no fanfare. Sharon and I lived with her family in order to save money while we were both in school. They provided a supportive environment for us.

My father died in the first year of my marriage to Sharon. He succumbed to several strokes over a relatively short period of time. Jane called my mother to tell her. My mother asked my younger brothers if they wanted to go to the funeral. Jane was told that they didn't want to go. I was saddened by this. I was certain that they would want to pay their final respects to our father. Jane and I went. I had only been to one other funeral, my grandfather's. That was a sad occasion. It was well attended. The car procession was long. I imagined It would be the same at my father's funeral. I was wrong.

My father's funeral was the saddest event I have ever attended in my life. He had six children, only Jane and I were there. There were maybe thirty people there, many of them church members. Aside from the family car, there were maybe three other cars in the funeral procession. I didn't shed a tear until I sat in the car next to Jane. I was suddenly struck by the fact that my father had lived a life where almost no one came to honor him. Four of his kids did not. Several family members did not.

I now view a funeral as a referendum one's life. People may not come to social events, but a funeral has a unique way of bringing people together. Attendance at a funeral often is visible statement about the impact that the person who has passed away has had on people. My father did not leave a significant impact. I never knew my father in an intimate sense. What I did know was that the people who knew him best decided not to attend his funeral. That was why I cried. Whenever I see a long funeral procession today I recognize the impact that person had on others. During my father's funeral, I vowed that although I had no children at that time, I would love my kids in such a way that they would all attend my funeral.

Although I struggled with the life lessons I learned in the aftermath of my father's death, I focused on a career in medicine. I graduated with honors from the Community College of Philadelphia with an Associate Degree in Applied Science. I minimized the importance of that achievement and didn't even attend my own graduation. I transferred to Saint Joseph's University to continue my education. Like many Pre-med students, I majored in Biology. I made the Dean's list in my first year, which was my third year of a four-year program. After taking the Medical College Admission Test, I was now ready to apply to medical school.

I had no confidence that I would be accepted to medical school. I had no one in my family to confide in. I was the first person to graduate from high school. By attending college, I had greatly exceeded the academic achievements of everyone in my family. This made me an oddity. I believed that my mother and Gene tried to discourage me. I was disappointed that there was no one to encourage me. Sharon and her family were kind to me but there was no praise from them either. This all fed into the narrative of my life. I had always done well in school, much better than my siblings but no one ever acknowledge my good grades as a kid. I wasn't surprised that it was the same now that I was an adult. I had internalized that experience to such an extent that I didn't revel in them either.

I applied to ten medical schools hoping that at least one would accept me. My first acceptance was to the now defunct Medical College of Philadelphia. My second acceptance was from Temple University School of Medicine. Temple University was my first choice for two reasons. The first reason was since I had worked at Temple University Hospital for years, I knew many of my coworkers would be happy for me. I knew it make them proud see me during my clinical years. I had fond relationships with many of the people I had worked with. Unlike my family, they genuinely supported me with their many words of encouragement. I knew they would be happy for me in a way that my family never would. The second reason was that it would vindicate me for my failed semester in 1979. I was eventually accepted by all eight schools who interviewed me. I decided to attend Temple University School of Medicine.

Medical school was a difficult adjustment for me. I had, what I thought, was a successful method of studying during my undergraduate years. I was overwhelmed by the sheer volume of information I had to master. Undaunted, I did my best. I thought that since I was successful as an undergraduate, I would be equally successful in medical school. I was not. I was an average student. This was a crushing blow to my ego because I was used to excelling when I gave a full effort. My foundation was shaken. The first two years of medical school I had to digest so much information, I wasn't sure I was going to survive medical school. I had to make sense of my predicament I developed the following analogy: students who are accepted to medical school are a select group. Not everyone who applies is accepted, the exceptional applicants are. I viewed acceptance to medical school was like being drafted into the NBA, your abilities are what gains you entry, and not everyone is LeBron James. Not everyone's name is known worldwide; their highlights are not shown on ESPN. They are still a NBA player. I decided not to rob myself of the fact that I had been accepted to medical school. I had earned my position there.

My clinical years in medical school had the greatest impact on my life. I was always a shy person. I was comfortable with that fact. In my clinical years, I was forced to come out of my shell. Before medical school no one had ever wanted my opinion about anything. I was good at regurgitating information, but analyzing and synthesizing information and then defending my thought process on the spot, was foreign to me. In the past I would fall back and let someone else take the lead. But now we each had to take turns taking the lead.

I had to show leadership skills during my clinical years to survive. There were many moments when I doubted myself. I would find, at my lowest moment, someone would encourage me. It was easy to tell that I was a medical student because I like all medical students wore a short white coat during our clinical rotations. At times I could feel a steady gaze on me. Usually it was an elderly person. A person who could have been my one of my grandparents would look me in the eye and say, "I am so proud of you." The first time it happened, I dismissed it, but it happened so many times that I couldn't helped but be encouraged.

In the clinical years of medical school, we had the opportunity to experience many specialties in medicine. The purpose was to broaden my knowledge base and to determine what field to choose for my career. Of all my clinical rotations, I enjoyed psychiatry the most but initially decided on anesthesiology because it was a more lucrative field. After graduation I felt I had a good chance of being accepted into Temple University Hospital's department of Anesthesiology since I'd worked there as an anesthesiology technician and I had a good relationship with the department chairman. I quickly found out there was a huge difference between my experience as a fourth-year medical student and an anesthesiology physician in-training, also called a resident. I struggled mightily and decided that anesthesiology was not for me. I decided to study what I truly enjoyed, psychiatry.

I don't know why I decided to go to the movies to see *Silence of the Lambs* a week before I started my psychiatry training. I remember watching Anthony Hopkin's thrilling portrayal of the main character, the murderous Hannibal Lecter. I was fascinated by Dr. Lecter's psychiatric acumen. I hoped that I would be able develop similar clinical skills as Dr. Lecter despite the fact he was a fictional character. I was amazed at how believable Anthony Hopkins was in that role. I was even more intrigued at his portrayal as the murderous Hannibal Lecter. I was almost certain that he would kill me before the end of the movie. I was plagued with the thought that the facility Hannibal Lecter was being treated in was like all psychiatric hospitals. I questioned if I was truly suited for a career in psychiatry. What would I do if I had to treat a patient like Hannibal Lecter? Lucky for me, I was mistaken. Psychiatry was much more manageable than what was depicted in *Silence of the Lambs*.

It is a commonly held belief that many people pursue a career into the mental health field to understand their own pathology. I can't speak for other mental health professionals, but that was true for me. During my psychiatry residency, I knew I had made the right choice. I noticed early in my training how people with mental illness and substance abuse issues were almost invisible to the rest of society. I could see the heartache and pain in the eyes of new admissions as they became acclimated to the inpatient unit. I understood how they felt. They were shocked that I would engage them in conversation. They thought I would treat them as if they were invisible. I knew how they felt. I often felt invisible within my own family. I always made a point of personally engaging the people under my care by acknowledging their humanity.

It was important that my patients be treated with dignity and compassion. I had the pleasure of being supervised on the inpatient unit by Dr. Louis Harris, an exceptional psychiatrist. He was knowledgeable and treated his patients with respect. He also taught me the value of observation. It was important for Dr. Harris to learn as much as he could about his patients. He valued the perspective of everyone involved in the treatment team, which included psychologists, nurses, psychiatry residents, mental health workers, and medical students. He considered all reasoned observations with equal weight.

I began to enjoy the attention I was receiving as a psychiatry resident. The nurses and support staff valued my easygoing demeanor. They praised me for it and that praise became intoxicating to me. I had not been exposed this level of affection in my life. It helped me don the mask of Dr. Jones. I started to actively behave in a manner to produce their adulation. Dr. Harris was clear about what he expected of me as a resident and it served to give me balance. He provided me with a good foundation in psychiatry. He was supportive of me, but was not one to overly praise the residents he trained. The staff on the inpatient unit, on the other hand, appreciated anyone who would acknowledged them as people rather than helpers to make the doctor's lives easier. I would address them respectfully and they appreciated it. I would also avoid conflict with them in order to be favored by them. I became self-deprecating. It became more important to be liked by the staff than to be forceful with my opinions.

I felt reborn. I was no longer Hurt Burt; I was Dr. Jones. Everybody liked Dr. Jones. I wore this mask because it did not allow my lack of self-esteem and lack of confidence to show. I had to be happy. Happy people attract people. I used humor around people. I enjoyed my status as Dr. Jones. It became important for me to endear myself to people and that everyone liked me. I would often exert a lot of energy to win people over. Even after I completed my training I strove to be popular among the support staff. I did not feel the same way about my peers. I wanted them to respect me but I kept them at a distance because I thought they might see through my façade.

Besides the accolades I received, I also enjoyed the money. I was used to a childhood of deprivation. I was used to delayed gratification. It was a way of life for me. When I became a doctor I suddenly had a significant increase in my income. I was not prepared for that. Instead of thinking about responsible things to do with the money, I started a pattern of conspicuous consumption. I wanted a nice car and some fancy clothes. Sharon and I thought about buying a big house. Instead of living within my means, I was creating this new persona. I was now fully Dr. Jones. He was going to be different from Burt. He was going to have the finer things in life. I was carefully crafting a mask that would cover the pain from the hurting child within me. I thought I could outdistance my past.

The transformation to Dr. Jones was quite an intoxicating experience. The kind words I received were shocking to hear initially since I grew up in a childhood where kind words were never spoken. I tended to behave in a manner that was not always true to myself. I was overly kind to people to elicit praise. I would find novel ways to ingratiate myself with others, for example if someone was selling candy bars for their child for a dollar a piece and their expectation was that I would buy five, I would buy twenty. I would then give the candy bars away thus magnifying my praise. It was very important that everyone liked, no, loved Dr. Jones. I was aware back then about how little I liked myself. It was through the perpetual praise of others that I started to think that I must be okay.

I wasn't a good steward of the money I earned. I wasn't making payment on my student loans. I wasn't always paying my full share of taxes. I was living a life that at times was more like a fantasy. The gnawing pain of abuse and neglect I faced as a child had seemingly disappeared. Instead of being dejected I felt happy. I thoroughly enjoyed going to work and it became like a drug to me. I was being praised for being nice to people and I was making a lot of money. Those things fed my fragile ego. I started spending more time at work than at home. There was a period of time when I worked about three years straight with one vacation day. It didn't bother me. I had no idea at the time how that imbalance would later impact my life.

Soon the simple adulation of staff was not enough. Since I was spending so much time at work, I began to have wandering eyes for the women there. The first time I had an affair, I battled within myself. I knew it was wrong but I enjoyed the attention. I ended the first affair after a few months and told Sharon about my transgression. She was devastated. I felt ashamed. We attended a marriage counseling conference at our church and that seemed to help. I left that job and hoped I had put that sordid event in my past. But within a few years I had two other brief affairs. I wanted to keep them a secret since I had cultivated such a positive image. I grew distant from Sharon. I was more focused on my life as Dr. Jones than being a husband and a father. I decided I wanted to be Dr. Jones full-time. I decided to separate from Sharon and I blamed her for my transgressions. This of course was not true. I deceived myself. Although I knew my leaving could have a negative impact on our four children, our daughters who were 8, 9, and 12 years of age our son was 15 years-old. I rationalized it by saying that since I was hardly home and worked so many hours, they wouldn't miss me. I was wrong and I would have to deal with that issue later.

It is written in Luke 12:3 (NIV), "What you have said in the dark will be heard in the daylight, and what you have whispered in the ear in the inner rooms will be proclaimed from the roofs." This came to life when I fathered a child with a woman I was having an affair with. My mask was starting to crack. I was more worried about my fractured reputation than wondering how to take care of the child once he was born. A darkness fell on my soul. I felt like people were whispering about me behind my back even though I couldn't prove it. Everyone seemed pleasant to me, however, I couldn't help but feel like they were looking at me with judgmental eyes. My son Camronn was born on February 28, 2006. I moved into this new phase of my life. I told Sharon about him even though we were separated at the time I felt she should know. I had expected her to become irate, she was not. She was supportive. I then told my children and they were bewildered. Their faces seemed to shout several questions. How did this happen? Who was his mother? What does this mean for us? This was the beginning of a severe fracture in my relationship with them, I was no longer the father they thought they knew. I had tarnished their image of me. They, however, fully embraced my son. They loved him from the first time they saw him. In many ways Camronn's loving smile and warm personality kept us united.

The fractured Dr. Jones persona finally died on Thursday June 29, 2006. I was called into my medical director's office and I was asked if I had any problems with my student loans. I said I knew I had defaulted on them and was planning to get on a payment plan. This was not true, but I felt that I had to tell them something. To be honest, I didn't care about paying my student loans at that time. I figured I would get around to it sometime in the future. At that moment, I found out that the future was now. Since I had defaulted on my federal student loans, I was placed on an exclusion list barring me from participating in the Medicaid/Medicare program until I paid the debt in full. What that meant was that I was not allowed to work at any facility that received Medicaid or Medicare funding. Furthermore, private insurance carriers would not provide payment for individuals who could not participate in the Medicaid/Medicare programs. I had four jobs at the time. Three of them received

Medicaid/Medicare funding. I lost all three of them at once. I had one consulting job that I could keep. It was the lowest paying of all of them. I immediately fell into a deep depression.

I thought that this would be easily remedied. After all the United States Department of Justice who handled my loan would surely want me employed as soon as possible to repay the debt. After I'd failed to respond to several of their letters, they were no longer interested in a quick resolution. I had lost that option. They wanted the entire $120,000 that I owed them which I did not have. I guess they assumed I was responsible with the money I was earning. This was not the case. At best I had maybe $2,000, which I now needed to live on.

Before this I never had any trouble sleeping. I was now plagued with insomnia. I spent many nights crying. I blamed myself for not being more responsible. I had placed my family in financial peril. I was flooded with the shame and guilt I had felt during my childhood abuse. I no longer had the mask of Dr. Jones to wear. I was devastated. My entire identity was tied to my Dr. Jones persona. Until that point of my life, I felt that I was well thought of by most people. Now I was sure I was the subject of ridicule. I had the scandal of a child out of wedlock and now I could not work in most of the jobs I had. I knew that many of my co-workers wondered why I wasn't working.

I heard that the rumor was that I lost my medical license. This was not true, but I guess it fit the narrative of someone whose life appeared to be out of control. When I wasn't working my consulting job, I would hide in my apartment. I was too ashamed to be seen in public. What could I say to people? My daily fear was when I went to my consulting job they too would tell me I couldn't work there but luckily, they never did. I believe it was God's providence that enabled me to keep that position.

Money was an issue for me during that time. I had grown accustomed to purchasing tailor made pants and expensive shirts. I would eat fancy meals. I drove a silver Mercedes Benz coupe. Now I had barely enough money to pay my bills. I had to provide support for my children who were suffering emotionally because of my separation from their mother. I ate less in order that they had enough to eat. I could no longer afford to take my clothes to be dry-cleaned. I wore only machine washable clothes. I had to park my Mercedes Benz because I didn't have enough money for gas, maintenance or auto insurance. I had to cash in my retirement fund to support my family. The first time I took public transportation was a humbling experience. I would always scan the crowd for anyone that I might know so I could avoid them. After all, why would Dr. Jones need to take the bus or subway, he had that big Mercedes Benz? I fell into a deeper depression, I wanted to believe that this was all a terrible nightmare. I hoped I would wake up and I would have more money in my pocket and I would jump into my fancy car and head off to work. Instead I would wake up and stare into the face of despair.

The worst feeling I had to deal with was to wake up and have nowhere to go. I went to my consulting job from 1:00 PM to 3:00 PM. I would wake up around 7:00 AM and could not go back to sleep, so I sat in a near fetal position until I had to go to work. I lead a very sheltered existence. I had very little contact with my mother or my siblings. We never talked about our struggles and this time was no different. I would get calls from the few friends that I had, but I wouldn't answer or return them. Each day was a painful burden. It was in that moment I became aware of my pain. Unlike the low level of pain, I usually dealt with, this was very different.

The usual pain I had to deal with I understood. I was a victim of childhood abuse and I felt damaged. I had an explanation for my feelings of low self-esteem. It was due to what I felt my mother and Gene had done to me. This pain was far different. It was from what I had done to myself. There was no way I could connect this to the past. I wanted to blame Sharon, but that did not ring true. In the abyss of my pain I had to first accept that I was responsible for the situation I was in. The tears I cried. The pain I felt was unbearable. I could feel the despair in my bones. It made me painfully aware of the present. I could not focus on the past. I had to muster up the strength to master the day.

I dealt with my pain day by day. I slowly learned to enjoy the little things like the food I ate as I started my day. I also enjoyed the gospel music I listened to on my iPod while I rode the bus and subway to work. After getting to work, I appreciated the warm greetings I received. At my consulting job, I completed court ordered psychiatric evaluations at the Criminal Justice Center, now called the Justice Juanita Kidd Stout for Criminal Justice, on Filbert Street. We affectionately called it the CJC. There were three people there who I counted on to get me through the day.

There was Linda Graham, a faithful Christian woman who always talked about her church, Enon Tabernacle Baptist Church. She was an administrative assistant in the mental health office at the CJC. She loved Jesus and she loved her church. But she wasn't a bible thumper, there was something real about her faith. She would often brag about her pastor. She told me he was an anointed preacher. Linda told me her church had made a gospel CD and her pastor Dr. Alyn E. Waller was featured on it. One day she brought me a copy of the CD. She asked me to listen to it. I thought I would hear the gravely tones of an old father of the church who on the recording would sound horrible. I had the experience in the past where those types of performance were best experienced live when you could feel the presence of the Holy Spirit. This was not the case as Pastor Waller had a wonderful booming voice that radiated with his love for God. I decided that one day I would visit her church.

Another person was Juanita Copeland, another one of the administrative assistants. Her warm smile comforted me when I arrived at the office. Before my situation, Juanita and I would exchange corny jokes about silly things at the office—a defendant who acted out, or something in the news. It didn't take much. During those days, I looked forward to our interactions. Her infectious laugh lifted me out of the pit of sadness I was in at least briefly. I can still hear that laugh even now.

Finally, there was William Washington, or Wash as he liked to be called. He was one of the sheriffs who would place the defendants in the holding cells for me to interview. He was a seasoned man who enjoyed life. He always greeted me with a strong hand shake and a warm smile. Before he'd place the defendants in the room, we would often chat. He would talk about his love for his wife or his struggles with the job. He always had a smile for me. He would often correct the other younger sheriffs and some of the defendants if they called me "Mr. Jones" instead of "Dr. Jones". At this period in my life, I was so sad that I never bothered to correct them. I didn't mind, but Wash did. "He's Dr. Jones. He worked hard for that.," Wash would say with a measure of assertiveness. In the shadow of my sadness, I walked in his support. It was sunshine to me.

When I got home I would spend hours on the telephone with a dear friend, Susan. Susan was a woman I was attracted to at one of the jobs I'd lost. I was interested in her but I don't think she was interested in me. Before I lost my job, I would ask her out. Sometimes she would say yes, sometimes no. I was separated from Sharon and that was an issue for her and rightfully so. I would often call her and we would have brief five to ten minute conversations. I was infatuated with her. I wasn't so sure she was with me. If I called her too often she would become upset and would end the call. This would hurt my feelings. Those interactions would tap into familiar feelings of low self-esteem, feelings I tried to hide under my mask. I would then not call her for a while. I would try to move on but I would continue think about her. After a few weeks, she would call me. I was excited when she did, only to ride a roller coaster of emotions with her. This on again off again relationship was something I could not understand, but I did not want it to end.

I never understood why she would talk to me for hours at a time back then. I know that I looked forward to our conversations. Those talks were about the events of the day. There was never any tension. She was expecting her first child and was in a committed relationship. She didn't know what to expect as a new parent. I shared my experience as a father. Our conversations provided a meaningful distraction for me during a dark period of my life. I would share bits of my childhood. I would talk about the abuse in an emotionally distant manner, as if it was something that happened years ago that I had dealt with it successfully. On a conscious level, I believed that. I felt she valued our talks then, in a way she hadn't in the past when we worked together. I couldn't explain it but I knew it was different. She was emotionally supportive of me. I needed that support. Our relationship existed only on the telephone. There were no dates. I valued her friendship. I believed that she valued mine. It was soothing to my soul. I learned a valuable lesson back then. In life, we may have many associates but very few friends. Susan was a friend.

I remember watching the movie *The Pursuit of Happyness*, starring Will Smith and his son Jaden Smith. It was about a father struggling through a period of poverty while maintaining custody of his young son and working at an unpaid internship. He struggled to be the best intern to hopefully obtain a lucrative job. His struggle to care for his son mirrored my struggle. He faced indignity after indignity. At the end of the movie, he was at his breaking point and had given up all hope of getting the job, but he got it.

Watching Will Smith find out that he got the job in the final scene was powerful. His tear soaked eyes showed both the fatigue of the struggle he survived and a tinge of disbelief. He then walked among a crowd who pay no attention to him while he expresses unbound joy. That scene touched me and when I first saw it, I openly wept. I felt his pain. I too was feeling the weight of my predicament. I was hoping that at the end of my journey, I too would be consumed by that same joy.

After months of corresponding with the United States Department of Justice, I was able to establish an agreement. I was overjoyed. I thought that I would quickly return to my old jobs and everything would be back to normal. I would experience happiness like Will Smith in the movie. That was not the case. I found out that I needed to reapply to participate in the Medicaid/Medicare programs. That was a time-consuming process that had to be done before I could be employed. After doing that, I found out that none of the hospitals where I was previously employed had a position for me. They had to move on and had filled my positions.

The first institution that hired me was Gaudenzia, Inc. Gaudenzia was well known in the Philadelphia area for its commitment to helping individuals struggling with drug and alcohol use. Although I had provided psychiatric support for people with substance abuse issues, it had always been in a setting where the focus was primarily on their mental illness. While mental illness was addressed in the residential program I worked in, there was much more support for recovery from substance abuse than I had been previously been exposed to. What impressed me was how we treated the people we helped. Hugs were common. The sharing of mutual experiences was honored.

I was taken aback by the experience because it spoke to me in a way that working in a primarily psychiatric setting had not. In those places psychiatric care was provided in a sterile fashion were boundaries were sacrosanct. While I understood theoretically why boundaries in general were important, and why some needed to be in place, for instance sexual relations with those under one's care and accepting of material gifts. But a hug of support, at times seemed important for both the person receiving the care and the person providing it. It acknowledged the humanity in them both.

Although I have never struggled with drugs or alcohol, I felt a certain kinship with the participants in recovery that I hadn't during my previous work experiences. Their stories of struggles with poverty resonated with me. The shame of having to do without was familiar to me. I was accustomed to always having a few dollars in my pocket. I now had maybe a few cents on a good day. I didn't always have enough food. This experience harkened back to my childhood. It was funny how I had forgotten those struggles.

I ate with the residents of the program. While I enjoyed sharing a meal with them and they enjoyed sharing a meal with me as well. I knew it would be my main meal of the day. I was self-conscious of the clothes I wore. I began work at Gaudenzia during the summer of 2007 and I would often sweat while taking the bus to work and I worried that someone would smell that my clothes needed to be sent to the dry cleaner. I thought I heard faint whispers about that. I was sure that there was whispers of things I'd done in the past. Those whispers echoed in my head. I may not have struggled with drugs or alcohol, but I did struggle with pain the way the residents in the program did. The embarrassment of past events weighed heavily on me.

EARLY ONE MORNING

During this journey, I had to turn back to my Christian faith.

I can clearly remember the day that Jesus came into my life. In the beginning of this book I shared with you the first time I invited Jesus into my life. I will now elaborate on that experience. He came by the invitation of a trembling, badly bruised, six-year-old boy. I was nibbling on a bit of food I'd snuck into my room. Even though Gene had forbidden it, I never felt comfortable eating in the dining room. I was too close to his ranting and raving. I felt so much more comfortable in the sanctuary of my modest bedroom. There I could decompress and savor a crust of bread or a piece of meat I had stealthily placed in my pocket.

The night before Gene had beaten us with extension cords. I hungered for any form of comfort and this food would be it. I made it up to my room and was nibbling on the food when I heard my younger brother Carl say words that chilled my soul. "Oooh, Ima' tell Gene." He had caught me. Fear overwhelmed me as tears welled up in my eyes. I knew if he told Gene that I was sneaking food, I would get another beating. The thought of another beating after just having one the night before was too horrible to consider. I begged him not to tell Gene as we stood at the top of the steps. He wouldn't listen to me and giggled as he ran down the stairs. Frightened, I suddenly recalled how we had learned about Jesus on the few times my mother would take us to church when we lived in Newark. I knew we could pray to him when we needed help. I knelt, and tightly intertwined my fingers.

"Jesus, please help me." I prayed. "I can't take another beatin', My back and arms and legs are all lumped up. They still hurt me. Please don't let Carl tell Gene. I can't take another beating." Tears streamed down my face as I opened my eyes and looked at the sun dimly shining through the window at the top of the stairs.

I then stood up and hid behind the bannister as I strained to hear what was happening downstairs. I heard Carl whisper something to Gene then Gene whispered back. I couldn't hear what they were talking about but I knew it was about me. My heart raced because I was sure Gene was going to call me down for a beating. The whispers stopped. The silence that followed was unbelievable. First, I heard Gene laugh. I then heard him walk towards the second-floor stairs and he walked down them as he headed out the front door whistling.

I was filled with joy. It was a strange emotion. In that moment, I understood that Jesus was real and that He had just saved me from a beating. I didn't know how He did it, I just knew that He did. And He did it simply because I asked Him to. Though that prayer didn't stop future beatings, it saved me from a beating that more than likely would have been devastating for me both physically and psychologically than any other. It is not that the beatings I received did not leave me with psychological scars, they did, it is just that there was always a period of days or weeks between them, which allowed my body to heal. The emotional abuse, however, was constant. The damage to my ego was incalculable.

That moment started my relationship with Jesus. I can't say that I was saved at that time because I didn't understand the concept of sin. At that age, I believed in my basic goodness. I viewed Gene as evil. I took solace in the fact that I did not treat people like he did. Back then I thought that I needed Jesus only in extreme situations. I was waiting for a similar horrible situation to occur. It never happened. I simply adapted to new life. I adjusted to the abuse and relegated Jesus to the few times I would go to church.

My attendance at church as a child was primarily going to vacation bible school during the summer at the Holy Redeemer Church. My mother had bought a set of encyclopedias that contained a book of bible stories. I enjoyed reading the stories about Adam and

Eve, David and Goliath and the life of Jesus. I also appreciated around Christmas when there were stories about the birth of Jesus Christ. I felt that Jesus was always nearby.

As a teenager, I dated a young lady whose family regularly attended church. She insisted that I attend with her. Her family church was a Holiness church. The service would start off with members of the congregation talking about what God done for them the past week. I would listen and was confused by what they were saying. They were not talking about anything miraculous. They were thanking God for their job and their family. What unnerved me was how they would emotionally confess their love for God. I began to question my relationship with God. I mean, I loved Him, but I was not as emotional as they were.

God began to reveal himself to me through people. The first person I saw God transform was a guy I knew in high school whose name was George. George was a few years older than me. He was a muscular guy who played on the football team. At my high school Friday the 13th was called Freshman Day. It was a day when the seniors would look for diminutive freshman like me and they would assault and humiliate them. I usually hid from the seniors. I did witness the abuse they unleashed on my classmates. They would stuff freshman in trashcans and roll them down a hill. They would smack them in the head, and rip their shirts. George would be one on the main perpetrators. He had a haunting laugh that scared me.

A few years later, while I was standing in front of my house, I saw him walking down the street toward me. My heart raced. I was now a junior in high school and George had graduated two years earlier. It was frightening for me to see him walking down my street. I was afraid he was going to recognize me and haze me. He was just as muscular as he was in high school. I was hoping he would walk by me but he did not. He stopped to talk to me and what he said was shocking. He asked me if I knew about Jesus and I said that I did. He told me that Jesus saved him and that his life was changed. He had such a gentle spirit that I thought I was talking to an entirely different person. He would walk through my neighborhood a few more time and he would talk to me about his love for the Lord. I thought at the time that it was strange.

When I attended the Community College of Philadelphia, I met another person who demonstrated how God can change a person's life. Aaron had dated Carla who worked with me and

Sharon at the Chemistry lab at Community College of Philadelphia. Aaron and Carla eventually were married. Sharon and I stayed in touch with them. We were shocked to find out years later that Aaron had left Carla and their two young daughters because he became addicted to drugs. They had just bought a house and Carla was struggling to keep it. We hoped that their marriage would be restored. We also would visit with Carla to give her support. After a few years, Aaron and Carla were reconciled. Their marriage blossomed. Aaron had accepted Jesus in his life and was a changed man. He used to have a biting sarcastic sense of humor but was now a gentle caring man who wanted everyone to know the Lord like he did. He became so devoted to his family. He had a gentle way that was admirable.

George and Aaron made such a transformation in their lives I could clearly see that God was using them. I wanted that for myself as a young man. I started attending church regularly. I understood that I needed to accept the Lord Jesus Christ as my Lord and Savior. I believed that He died for my sins and was resurrected in three days with all power in His hands. I became aware of my own sin nature. I struggled with self-esteem issues. I knew I was not following what

God would want me to do. I struggled with bitterness and resentment that I attributed to my painful childhood. I confessed my sins to him. I was baptized by the late Reverend Daniel Clater at the 48th Street Baptist Church when I was twenty-two. I began to feel God's presence in my life, but not like it was for George and Aaron. I soon felt myself drifting away from God. Eventually I stopped attending 48th Street Baptist Church.

The Lord continued to tug on my heart. I decided that I needed to rededicate myself to the Lord. I needed to lead my family. Sharon and I, along with our two children at that time, joined Bethany Baptist Church. The Reverend Alpheus Bright was our pastor. The name Pastor Bright suited him because he had such a bright smile. His sermons of hope and redemption touched me. I loved the hug I received from him at the end of service. It took the place of the hugs I never got from my father or Gene. Pastor Bright put me to work at the church as a trustee. I enjoyed my time at Bethany. I still however felt a void between me and God.

I liked listening to hip-hop music and rhythm and blues at home. I would listen to hymns and spirituals at church. Over time I would find myself drawn to gospel music. I especially enjoyed listening to the choir sing the hymn *Blessed Assurance* and wanted to buy a cassette tape of it. There were no iPods back then, only the Walkman. Finding gospel music was difficult at that time, secular music was much easier to find. I was living in Southwest Philadelphia at the time. I found a record store not far away that had a copy of Daryl Coley's *In My Dreams* cassette and I loved it. He had a rendition of *Blessed Assurance* on it. I have been a fan of his music ever since. Kirk Franklin's debut album, Kirk *Franklin and the Family,* also had a huge impact on me. As I listened to each song on the album I started to cry. Other songs by other artist would also have that same effect. I was bewildered by this. No other genre of music had the same effect. I began to develop a fondness for gospel music.

I enjoyed going to church and learning about the bible. I started memorizing bible verses. Although I knew that attending to church was the right thing to do, I went sporadically during football seasons. I also sometimes found the sermons boring in stretches. At times, I even thought I was doing God a favor by attending. This is back when things were going great for me. I had graduated medical school and was making good money. I had a wonderful family and beautiful children. Most importantly, I thought, although I had a rough childhood, I was basically a good person. I ignored the sin nature I knew was within me.

Before long, my work began to take priority in my life. I would place God on the back burner. This set the stage for my adulterous affairs. The combination of the time I spent at work, the adulation I received there and my lack of commitment to the study of God's Word created enough distance between me and God where an affair was possible. After the initial effects of the first affair wore off, it was easier to have the next. I told myself that Sharon did not love me the way these other women did. I could not see my brokenness in any of it. Sometimes I would be racked with guilt. On those occasions I would justify my indiscretions by telling myself I had married too young. Since Gene never allowed me to have an active social life, I thought I was making up for lost time. Out of one of my liaisons came my youngest child, Camronn. Embolden by my brazen behavior, I asked Sharon for a divorce. She did not want a divorce. She wanted to remain married. Over time she relented, more than likely she wanted to spare our children from a bitter divorce battle.

I didn't seek the Lord's advice in this matter. I harbored guilt about how my children suffered. They always seemed to put on a good face for me when I went to see them. I would try to ease their pain by buying them gifts. That made me feel that I was active in their lives. I was so far from God at this stage of my life. I was making decisions I thought was in my best interest with little regard to how I was hurting my children. I was so blind.

Susan started to have a more prominent role in my life after my divorce. I eventually fell in love with her but I was not certain that she felt the same way about me. I asked God for a sign that she cared for me. Over a period of time she appeared to have an interest in me. We shared may conversations about significant past life events. I told her about my childhood abuse. As I talked about the past I had believed that I was heading to a happier life. I felt that I was distancing myself from my past. Susan eventually confessed her love for me and our relationship became important for the both of us. We were eventually married. Our marriage was rocky from the start. What neither one of us discussed or considered was how we were going to blend our new family. She had a child from a previous relationship and I had five children, four from Sharon—two late teen daughters as well as an adult daughter and son—and another son from a previous relationship. My older children tolerated Susan because of me: they each clearly preferred that I reunite with their mother. Susan, in turn, was superficially pleasant and emotionally distant from them. Camronn was well received by my children and Susan.

My relationship with my older kids became a source of stress for me and Susan. Susan felt that my kids would tie me to Sharon. I was placed in the awkward position of balancing loyalties to Susan and my kids. This was perhaps one of the most stressful times in my life. At times it seemed that no one was pleased with me. I would feel torn as I drove to visit my kids. I would often cry on the way home once I left them. Their pained expressions while I was there and the lingering hugs as I left, took their toll on me.

Susan and I had many arguments about how we could make our blended family work. Susan was loud at times and quite vocal. I, on the other hand, was quiet. Susan would raise her voice at me and I'd become quite numb and emotionless. Although I didn't recognize it in the beginning, this experience took me back to the times when Gene would yell at me before he'd beat me. I think I didn't allow myself to be in touch with my emotions because I didn't want to experience that level of fear again. I tried to think of words that would allow me to communicate my feelings, but none came out of my mouth. Some of Susan's words however, were quite biting. When I felt hurt, I would lash out verbally and we would end up hurting each other. We epitomized the phrase 'hurt people hurt people.' We tried marital counseling twice. Therapy may have slowed the frequency of our arguments, but not the ferocity. We decided to take a break from couple's therapy and sought individual therapy.

We decided to go on a trip for our third anniversary. During the trip, we had another heated argument. I went into the bathroom of our hotel room and had a meltdown. I turned on the faucet to muffle my tears. I felt overwhelming fear. It was like I was a young child again. I was scared, trembling in fear, wondering what would happen next. I wanted to run and hide. I was at my wit's end. I knew I could no longer tolerate this feeling. I felt like I was having a nervous breakdown, and there was no one to comfort me. I had to get away to maintain what little bit of my sanity I had left. A few months prior to that trip, I had signed a lease for an apartment. I contemplated when would be the time to leave. After the argument at our trip, I felt that this was the time to leave. I did not consult God. The decision was made out of anger. Two weeks after we returned, I left Susan. She had no idea I was leaving. I had felt that I had enough of the arguing. I was never good at confrontations. Most of the time I would either suppress my feelings. Just like with Sharon, I ran away. I ran away again. I eventually told her by text as I was too angry at the time to tell her in person. This was not the best way to handle things, but I was fearful of another volatile confrontation. I had decided to leave in the summer because I didn't want to disrupt the children's—her daughter and my son's—school year.

The first three weeks after I separated from Susan I fell into a pit of depression. I had placed my hopes and dreams on a relationship that for all intents and purposes was over. I couldn't eat. I couldn't sleep. I cried all the time when I was in my apartment. I didn't know what to say to Camronn, he loved Susan and her daughter. This was almost as devastating to me as when I lost my job from the Medicare/Medicaid program in 2006. The major difference was I could talk to Susan then. This time I had no one to talk to. But I felt justified in my decision because of Susan's anger and the feelings it brought up in me. I thought she needed to do something about her anger. I processed some of my feelings with my therapist, but that didn't help me when I was back in my lonely apartment.

I tried to convince myself that it was Susan's fault that I had to leave. As the days flowed into weeks, I started to miss her. But how could I resolve this dilemma? I had arranged for my mail to be forwarded to a PO box. When I checked it, I saw I had a summons to appear in court. Susan was suing me for spousal support. I knew I would have to pay her spousal support, but I hoped perhaps we might get back together. But how could we, we hadn't spoken to each other in weeks? I decided to contact the attorney who handled my divorce from Sharon. I was starting to feel the weight of my situation. My life was falling apart, once again.

It was time to evaluate my life. I had one failed marriage and a current one that was failing. I had hurt my kids in the process. I hurt my kids the same way my father hurt me; I abandoned them. Although no one at work knew my personal situation, I bore the weight of shame as I carried out my duties. The whole world became varying shades of gray. Each day it was harder to act like everything was fine. I wanted to attend church but I didn't out of shame and embarrassment. I had no one to turn to. No one could understand me except one person, Jesus Christ. I knew I had tried to work things out myself, but I failed miserably. I realized that I wanted to restore my marriage. I prayed that Susan would get help for her problem with anger. I prayed and cried, prayed and cried. Then early in the morning of July 26, 2014, I heard the voice of the Lord clearly for the first time. It was the still small voice that Elijah heard in 1 Kings 19:12. God said to me that Susan wasn't the one who was angry, it was me.

It was then that the blinders of my reasoning fell away. I now understood exactly what God meant. I had not consulted His Word when I made the decision to leave Susan. I did not consult any church leaders for wise counsel. I didn't even get on my knees and talk to God about this decision. Out of anger I felt I had enough and decided to act on that emotion. I then had the audacity to ask God to change her, without once considering what needed to change in me. I wept loudly at that point. I was then compelled to contact Susan. It was about two o'clock in the morning so I decided to text an apology. I didn't expect a response. I didn't expect a response at all given what I had done.

I got up around 7:30 AM full of joy and a sense of relief. I thought I was beginning to put life back together. I called Susan to beg her forgiveness. She didn't answer so I left a voicemail. Despite that I felt boundless joy. I had never felt this way in my entire life. It was a wonderful gift from God. I went to church that morning with unbridled exuberance. For the first time, I truly had a song in my heart.

As I returned to my apartment, I received a call from Susan. I sensed an emotional distance between us. It didn't matter to me, I had an opportunity to express my feelings for her. I gave her a heartfelt apology. She listened to me. Her words seemed measured, as if she was protecting herself from me. She asked me where I was living and I told her. She said she would be right over. I was nervous once I hung up the telephone. I had not seen her more than three weeks. I didn't know how this meeting would go. I feared that it would end in an argument.

I felt buoyed by God's love for me. I rested on His strength. When I saw Susan outside my building she had the residue of pain in her eyes. She was silent as we shared the elevator ride to my apartment. I showed her around my sparsely decorated apartment.

She saw the inflatable bed I slept on. I had a television. There was no furniture. We sat on the floor and wept as we talked about how hard the past few weeks had been. We had a heartfelt conversation about our individual experiences. It was clear that we still loved each other. It was also clear that we knew our marriage needed work.

After a few weeks, we decided that we would seek marital counseling within our church. I called one of the pastors in charge of mental health support and asked if he would be willing to counsel us. He said that he would but he wanted us to read some information before we met with him. It was titled *What is God's Primary Purpose of Marriage?* It explained how God views marriage. What touched me was the explanation that love as an act and not only an emotion, as I thought it was. I realized that my love for Susan was a self-serving love. I should love my wife not because of what she does for me but because of what the Word of God says.

I had also harbored animosity toward Susan that I chose to ignore. I focused on her behaviors and responded to them in an emotional way. I did not consider how Jesus would handle our situation. I felt justified in my actions. There was no measure of forgiveness. I had convinced myself that I had forgiven her, I now realized that I put a limit on how much forgiveness I would extend her. I forgot how Jesus responded when asked by Peter in Matthew 18:21-22, many times we should forgive, seven times. Jesus replied seventy times seven. I figured I had forgiven her that 490 times Jesus said, even though I knew the scripture meant to always forgive. I needed to forgive her as Jesus forgave me. It was clear that I was not living out my faith.

I read in the information that we learn the most about Jesus through our marital difficulties. Through that suffering, I would have to turn to Christ for my strength. Initially, I thought I understood that. My comprehension at the time was merely superficial. There was so much weighty material I tried to digest in a few readings. I had deceived myself into believing that by reading and rereading I could grasp the deeper meaning of scriptures such as Hebrews 5:8 (KJV), "Though He were a Son, yet learned He obedience by the things which he suffered." And Zechariah 13:9 (KJV), "I will refine them like as silver is refined, and will try them as gold is tried: they shall call on My name, and I will hear them: I will say, it is my people: and they shall say, The Lord is my God." I eventually learned that with continued prayer, the deeper meaning of the scriptures would be revealed to me.

What I also learned from reading *What is God's Primary Purpose of Marriage?* was the difference between happiness and joy. I had spent my entire life in the pursuit of happiness. Never once did I consider the definition of happiness. Happiness is based on circumstances. Without a positive set of circumstances, there can be no happiness. Joy is different. Joy comes from trust in God's love and sovereignty. It is an inner peace not based on circumstance. It is the substance of what filled me up on July 26, 2014. I had never felt anything like it before.

I prayed more fervently than I ever had. I had a song in my heart and I was uplifted by it. I thought Susan and I were headed in the right direction. I read many books that were suggested to us like *The Power of the Praying Husband* by Stormie Omartian, *Hope for the Separated* by Gary Chapman, and *Forgiveness* by Iyanla Vanzant. These books were informative. I felt that I was renewing myself in the process.

I had a renewed dedication to my marriage. Even though we were still separated, I would mail Susan a card every day. The cards chronicled what the Lord had accomplished in my life that day. I also told her how much I loved her. We continued to meet with the associate pastor for marital counseling. He suggested that we attend a marital support group. It was initially helpful for us. We saw that we were not the only couple at our church struggling with marital issues.

We focused on working harder on our marriage, but I noticed that Susan was withdrawing somewhat from the process. She started to question my motives. My anger slowly began to eat into my joy. I decided to redouble my efforts. Instead of sending cards daily, I would send her a text messages the first thing in the morning. I enjoyed this ritual of love. However, over time old behaviors emerged. I felt irritable and started to withdraw when I didn't get the response I wanted. I wanted Susan to lovingly acknowledge my efforts. Instead Susan became harsh in her words. I selfishly interpreted that as anger instead of realizing that she was just as hurt as I was.

I was still seeing my therapist. He thought that perhaps our marriage was over. I told him that I was not interested in another divorce. I wanted to be true to God's Word in a way I had not been with my first wife. Despite some setbacks, I knew God would work it out for us. My therapist began to focus on Christian themes after my discussion of Christ's impact on my life. I thought our therapy was moving in the right direction.

Even though Susan and I had moments of tension, we still made time for each other. We would go out on dinner dates on the weekends when her daughter was with her father and my son was with his mother. This occurred every other weekend. On one weekend Susan wanted to watch the movie *Twelve Years a Slave*. I loathe movies about slavery. I was quite knowledgeable about the slave experience of my ancestors and did not enjoy watching depictions of the brutality associated with it. I felt I had seen enough of that through the *Roots* miniseries by Alex Haley and countless movies afterwards. One movie that turned me against watching such films was a movie that had a limited run. It was titled *Sankofa*, it was advertised by word of mouth in 1993. I don't think I had ever seen a movie with more graphic violence than that one. I was no longer interested in seeing that that kind of movie because it made me angry.

I decided that I would watch *Twelve Years a Slave* with Susan because she wanted to watch it as it was an Oscar contender. In the beginning of the movie, the title character was whipped as a way of indoctrinating him into a life of slavery. I had seen scenes like that in several movies. On that night instead of watching a man being whipped, I had a different experience. The whistle of the whip through the air sounded eerily like the extension cord Gene used to beat me with. The pitch of the sound of the striking his body was the same sound I heard when the extension cord struck my body. It was like I was being beaten. I felt the extension cord on my back and fear overwhelmed me. I bolted out of the room. I went upstairs and I noticed that I was trembling. The echoes of the snap of the extension cord played on what seemed like an endless loop. For the first time in my life I had a flashback. I wanted to tell Susan that night, but I couldn't. I had no words that could accurately express what I felt. I didn't know what to make of that experience. I needed to process it with my therapist. I did talk to Susan about it later. She said she noticed that it appeared something had upset me. She didn't know what to say to me. I don't what she could have said I was awe-struck.

When I went to see my therapist, I was oddly excited. For years, I struggled with depression and low self-esteem. I wondered if I suffered from Post-Traumatic Stress Disorder in the past but I thought my symptoms were closer to Dysthymia, which a mild form of depression. I could not ignore what had just happened. I had a moment of clarity. I thought after telling my therapist what happened, my therapy would start to focus on my traumatic past. Instead, my therapist simply listened to me. I waited for a few sessions to see if he would address the issue of trauma. He never did. During my last session, he gave me a homework assignment: I was to come up with a list of the three celebrities I most identified with and write why I chose them. I never completed the assignment and I never returned for therapy. I didn't see how that assignment addressed my current issue. What was the point?

ALONE

Back in October of 2014 I felt truly alone. I was still separated from my second wife. I had just terminated therapy. I knew I had recently suffered a flashback and didn't know what to make of it. I felt a distance from God. I was in the icy confines of loneliness. I went through the motions of the day. I can't say that I was sad as much as I felt that I was questioning my purpose. I began to look over the fabric of my life. I questioned the decisions I had made. I started to live a life of regret. I didn't know where to turn. I did the only thing I knew how to do and that was to get on my knees and pray. As I prayed I remembered the words of Daryl Coley's song, "I'll Be With You."

That song, as well as many others, demonstrates the transformative nature of gospel music. "I'll Be With You" speaks to the time I prayed to Jesus as a six-year-old and it continues to feed my soul ever since I first heard it in the early 1990s. It has helped me through the valley of despair. At that time, it ministered to me. It was as if Jesus was speaking to me through Daryl Coley's words. When I listen to gospel music I experience my Christian faith in a tangible way. I had a sense of what Daniel felt in the lion's den, what Shadrach, Meshach and Abednego felt in the fire, and what David felt before battling Goliath. Jesus was indeed with me.

I got up from praying and I started my journey toward healing. My previous attempts at therapy were not helpful but I was not willing to give up on it. As a psychiatrist, I was certain that therapy could be helpful. I knew that there was therapy for survivors of childhood trauma. During my residency I was taught and supervised in various forms of psychodynamic therapy. There was not a specific focus on helping individuals with the specific issue of trauma during my training. Throughout my career my focus was on performing psychiatric evaluations and medication management, not psychotherapy. I was now focused on finding information about treatment for PTSD and how it applied to me as well as the individuals I had the honor to treat.

As I coped with this feeling of being alone, I was often reminded of one of the many conversations I had with Laverne

Yeargins-Clark. She is a devout Christian and would often talk about her love for her husband and their children. She credits her faith to her late father, John Yeargins, the former pastor of Smith Chapel Church on 1825 Ridge Avenue. She would often share with me the many conversations she had with her beloved father. He had such a comforting relationship with God. Her father, preferred to live alone in his own home after her mother's death. Laverne would often call him and ask if anyone was with him. He would reply, "no, it's just me and Jesus." As I travel this road of solitude, I reflect on the words of this man who had such a deep faith. What took me several years to learn, Pastor Yeargins always knew: we are never alone because Jesus is always with us. I took comfort in that knowledge.

I reviewed the criteria for the diagnosis of PTSD in the Diagnostic Statistical Manual (DSM) fifth edition, commonly called DSM V. It is the book that contains the criteria for the diagnosis of all accepted and identified mental health concerns. PTSD, as classified in DSM V, is triggered by exposure to actual or threatened death, serious injury, or sexual violation. The exposure must result from one or more of the following scenarios, in which the individual:

A. Directly experiences the traumatic event.

B. Witnessed the traumatic event in person.

C. Learns that the traumatic event occurred to a close family member or close friend (with the actual or threatened death being either violent or accidental) or;

D. Experiences first-hand repeated or extreme exposure to aversive details of the traumatic event (not through media, pictures, television or movies unless work-related).

The disturbance, regardless of its trigger, causes clinically significant distress or impairment in the individual's social interactions, capacity to work or other important areas of functioning. It is not the physiological result of another medical condition, medication, drugs or alcohol.

The strict definition of PTSD did not quite reflect my history. My past consisted of episodes of chronic emotional abuse and neglect, intermingled with episodes of horrific physical abuse. Even though I had a recent flashback, I struggled trying to reconcile my experience with the definition in DSM V. In my search for answers, I discovered Dr. Judith Lewis Herman's phenomenal book, *Trauma and Recovery*. It is a must-read for anyone who wants to have a clear understanding of trauma and the issues involved in its treatment throughout the history of psychiatry. *Trauma and Recovery* discusses the history of the treatment of trauma from the early work of Dr. Sigmund Freud and her struggles to have clearer descriptions of types of PTSD in the current editions of the DSM. In her book, Dr. Lewis Herman discusses the political nature of the treatment of trauma survivors. It is through the era of the fight for women's rights and the need for treatment for Vietnam war veterans where survivors of all types of trauma were diagnosed and treatment was finally considered in a systematic fashion.

It was in her discussion of Complex PTSD that I began to understand myself better. Dr. Lewis Herman studied several individuals with this condition and presented her findings to the American Psychiatric Association to be included in DSM IV and V to no avail. What distinguishes Complex PTSD from PTSD in the chronic nature of the abuse under totalitarian control. She included in her findings, hostages, prisoners of war, concentration camp survivors and survivors of religious cults. She also included survivors of domestic battering, and childhood physical and sexual abuse.

There are many types of abuse. I experienced emotional abuse which involved the use of vulgar demeaning language which often included threats of violence. I also experienced physical abuse through the beatings I endured with the extension cords. There was also abuse through neglect, where nurturing was denied and my basic need for food and clothing was ignored. I never experienced sexual abuse. That type of abuse can have a devastating impact on a young child. It involves such an intimate betrayal. I would often minimize my experience because I was not sexually abused. What I came to realize was that I was not being true to my experience. I cannot minimize it. What happen to me was horrible and should not have happened, but, since it did, I must be honest about the devastating impact it has had on my life.

I read Dr. Herman's book with piqued interest. She put into words how isolated I felt as a young child. How I would demonize Gene, but give my mother a pass because I wanted to maintain a loving relationship with her. I never had such a relationship with Gene. One thing that rang true for me was Dr. Herman's discussion of the issue of self-blame. Throughout my life, beginning in early childhood, I would blame myself for things that didn't go as planned for me. Whether it was relationships with peers or competition during sport activities, if the outcome was negative, I blamed myself for it. I would redouble my efforts at the next opportunity. I would never call to mind successful interactions, only failures, thus I felt like I was always failing and thus the burden of blame became oppressive. I would minimize my successes such as my good grades and getting into medical school, since no one in my family made a big deal of them. I always felt like I was different in a way I could not understand. I placed a great deal of emphasis on being well-behaved in school and getting good grades to try to please Gene. None of that mattered. What did serve me well during my childhood was my belief in my own goodness. Later, it was that thought process would lead to my downfall.

What intrigued me the most about Complex PTSD was the concept of emotional flashbacks. I was aware that flashbacks, recurrent involuntary memories of past traumatic events, can be triggered by things you see, hear, taste, smell and feel. Psychologist Peter Walker in his book *Complex PTSD: From Surviving to Thriving* defines emotional flashbacks as intense disturbing regressions to feelings of being overwhelmed, as one was in childhood. While in the midst of a flashback, fear, shame, or depression can dominate your experience. That was an eye-opening revelation for me.

I had many heated arguments with Susan. When I became upset, I wanted to end the discussion, but Susan would persist. I had never been in a relationship where there was so much contention. Initially, I would try to see her point with the idea she would also consider mine. There were occasions she would, but for the most part she would press the issue to make her point. As I would get angry, my perception was that she was yelling at me. Many times, this was not the case. I would find myself frozen, physically and emotionally. It was as if I had shut down. Like a computer, I would switch to sleep mode. I had nothing to say. Inwardly, I felt ashamed as if I should have done something different or better. I had no idea I was tapping into the memories I had as child. It was if I were a young child again, standing in front of Gene. Oddly enough, I never had that experience with anyone else.

I wanted to understand how I could escape from this emotional quagmire I felt trapped in. I wanted to find my way out after accepting that I was a survivor of childhood abuse. I was ready to begin the process. Even though I realized that it may be difficult to start the discussion, I had many concerns about how I would feel as I went through the recovery process. I also wondered what that process would proceed. In *Trauma and Recovery*, Dr. Herman outlines the process of recovery as falling into three basic stages. She states these stages are not a continuum from one to the next, but as processes that help to make a person whole. The first stage is safety, the second stage is remembrance and mourning and the third stage is the reconnection with ordinary life.

Before the first stage can be addressed, the condition of PTSD must be identified. This resonates with me because I could not, or would not, have discovered my diagnosis without identifying my symptoms. It was important for me to seek support once I knew what the focus of my treatment should be. Throughout my life, I never truly felt that I had a sense of self. That was why the persona of Dr. Jones had been so important to me. Since recent life experiences had removed that from me I truly felt lost. I was now in pursuit of finding out who I truly was. I didn't feel safe in my world, not even safe in my own skin.

In determining safety, Dr. Herman talks about removing yourself from the toxic environment that abuse thrives in. I thought that happened when I was kicked out of my childhood home. It provided a relative moment of safety for me at the time. As I look back on my first marriage to Sharon, I floated through that experience feeling numb. I was emotionally distant from Sharon and my children. I even felt alone when I was in a room with them. However, as Dr. Jones, I was thrilled with the interactions I had with people at work. My life as a husband and a father seemed boring in comparison. I became disenchanted with my first marriage. Marital infidelities on my part led to our divorce. I thought that I was free to pursue my own happiness with little regard to the emotional wake I had created. Sharon and my children were devastated and I didn't consider their feelings at all.

Nevertheless, I proceeded with my illusory pursuit of happiness. I needed to redefine myself. I wanted to learn from the mistakes I'd made in my first marriage. After I fell in love with Susan. I wanted to have a second chance of having a committed relationship. I had no idea just how difficult it was to manage a blended family. I was pulled in two directions: in one direction from my kids and in another from Susan. I felt that when I was with one, I was betraying the other. Susan and I would often argue about the time I spent visiting my kids. What I had become blind to, was the toxic environment created for me by my second marriage.

During the early years of our marriage, Susan would berate me whenever she became upset. She would want to have discussions, but I would avoid them because her nonverbal communication demonstrated to me that she was angry. I knew that if she was angry it would be impossible for me to be heard. To be clear, she had valid points, it was her delivery of those points that wounded me at my core. When I tried to communicate this to her, she was not able to hear me. This set the stage for a dance of toxic shame for me. I would try to weather the storm of her verbal tirades unaware, in the beginning, that I was experiencing emotional flashbacks. All I knew was that I felt strange, as if I were floating while feeling overwhelming fear.

I often wondered, even while I was separated from Susan why was I still so attracted to her. At first I thought the attraction was physical since she was and still is quite attractive. I thought it had to be deeper than that and as I pondered Dr. Lewis Herman's book, I could understand the unconscious thoughts that I was initially blind to. Susan represented to me an amalgam of my mother and Gene. I loved and loathed her at the same time. My love for her always seemed stronger. Susan would tap into my animosity for Gene whenever we argued. Those feelings would become so intense that I would not speak to her for days even though as a Christian I knew the Bible states in Ephesians 4:26 (KJV) "Be ye angry, and sin not: let not the sun set on your wrath." I struggled mightily with that verse.

I felt a sense of uneasy calm between arguments. I was afraid to say anything, fearful that anything I'd say would propel us into the next argument. I felt the same way as a young child around Gene. I also yearned to receive from Susan the same validation I had wanted from my mother but never received. I would constantly rethink my past actions. I would try different approaches to show her how much I loved her only to have my attempts thwarted. I would still try to seek her approval and never felt I achieved it. It was eerie when I think of how similar this was to my relationship with my mother. Ultimately, I felt I had to separate from Susan to feel safe. I thought I was running away from her: instead I found out I was trying to run away from my past.

Dr. Lewis Herman writes that the establishment of self-care can be quite complicated for survivors of trauma because it is a skill many have not put into practice Survivors avoid standing out in their environments and find it hard to act against those individuals who have harmed them. It is important to give support to survivors so they are able make a decision that is in their best interest and not allow others to force to take a plan of action against their will. Self-care can be quite difficult for childhood abuse survivors because many may be engaging in self-harming behavior such as chronic suicidality, self-mutilation, eating disorders, or acts of sexual abuse. These activities serve to modify what is often unacceptable feelings in the absence of alternative methods to manage unwanted feelings. My ability to care for myself was thwarted by the negative self-talk I engaged in. I was far more critical of myself that anyone else was of me.

Dr. Lewis Herman also mentions that the establishment of safety can become a battle on two fronts by the client against the therapist. On one front, the client may be so consumed with self-hatred that it is difficult for them to accept that therapy as something they are worthy of. On the other hand, the client who prefers to be invested in the fantasy of being rescued may resent the work and want the therapist to do it. It is vital, at this stage, to discuss the issue of client safety and who will be responsible for it.

I believe that it is my responsibility to develop the skills necessary to maintain my own safety. To accomplish this, I felt I had to separate from Susan to create an environment where I could focus inward with minimal distraction when I was at home. In that time alone however, I spent a lot of time criticizing my past actions. It was helpful that I had also began treatment with a new therapist. I was interested in renewed focus with my therapy. I also spent more time praying for God's guidance. I learned through my bible study just how much work I had to do. The Lord revealed to me where I fell short of His Word. This was a humbling period in my life. I was holding myself responsible for my actions in a way that I never had.

Dr. Mario Martinez, in his book, *The Mind-Body Code*, talks about how the way we think affects how our body responds to stress. He states that establishing safety is needed to work through fear. The feeling of safety can be achieved by how we position our body. He suggests that we sit in chair, or edge of a pillow with our legs uncrossed and our feet on the floor. Or we can have our back against a wall or a chair. If chair is used, let it support the weight of your body, this reduces stress. Then take slow relaxing breathes through your abdomen, breathing through any tension you sense in your body. When I performed his exercises, I began to develop a sense of relief. Dr. Martinez's audio book series provides thoughtful explanations of his theories in a far more detailed fashion than is discussed here and you should refer to his book for more detailed information about this technique.

Dr. Lewis Herman's second stage of recovery is remembrance and mourning. This is the stage where the story of the trauma is discussed completely and in depth with as much detail as possible. The telling of the story in its entirety can be transformative. It should be done at the client's own pace. The choice to confront these horrors rests with the survivor. This is the stage where careful detailed work can be done. The pace should be decided by the survivor with the therapist providing support and working as an ally in this process. Dr. Lewis Herman states that it is important for the survivor to reconstruct the story before the trauma began. This serves to recreate the flow of one's life before the trauma to restore a sense of continuity with the past. There should be, if possible, a discussion of goals and ambitions before the trauma to establish a context for how the trauma impacted them. The next step is to reconstruct the traumatic events as a statement of fact. This creates a narrative that includes the survivor's response to it as well as the responses of the important people during that time. Some of the events may not be easily expressed in words, but may be expressed nonverbally through drawing or painting. It is important to have a complete narrative that includes vivid details. It is also vital that a description include all five senses. It should include what was heard, seen, smelled, felt and even tasted. It is difficult work, but it is necessary, as these dark secrets are the essence of what holds the survivor back from truly appreciating life in the present. During this stage, it is crucial to ensure the survivor can maintain a sense of safety during this difficult, and, at times, frightening work. The therapist must serve as a steady reassuring presence during this process.

As I moved into this stage, it was indeed quite frightening. I had suppressed the horrible memories of my abuse. As I told my story to my EMDR therapist, I was transported back to my childhood home. The worst memories were the many times we were all lined up shoulder to shoulder. I could feel the coldness of the dimly-lit room. I experienced the smell of mothballs and plaster. I felt waves of panic as I waited my turn to feel the burning sting of the extension cord. I hadn't consciously thought about that time in my life in decades. It was amazing how emotionally charged just thinking about it was. It, however, was important for me to face those memories.

There are losses associated with trauma. Survivors who may have endured physical trauma often struggle with the psychological loss of the self. They may also have to cope with the loss of the feeling that their body is their own. There is a mourning that is different from that of an important person, these losses are invisible or unrecognizable. The usual means of mourning do not provide comfort. As I reflect on my life, I realize, I hadn't had a sense of self since the time I lived in Newark.

Mourning can be difficult and survivors may create ways to avoid it. One of those ways is the revenge fantasy. This is a mirror image of the traumatic event where the roles of the perpetrator and victim are reversed. The survivor in this instance believes that revenge is the only way to restore lost power. Revenge only serves to keep the survivor in emotional turmoil as it causes a reliving of the trauma. The survivor must realize that revenge only leads to an increase in experience of torment. Another alternative way of putting off mourning is the what Dr. Lewis Herman calls the fantasy of forgiveness. She believes that true forgiveness can only be achieved when the perpetrator has sought and earned it through confession, repentance and restitution.

As a Christian, I disagree with this characterization of forgiveness. For a Christian, forgiveness is required whether the injured person has received an apology or not from the person who has caused the injury. Forgiveness first is for the survivor and is then extended to the perpetrator. Christ is our model. When we were sinners He died for us. We are to be conformed into His image, and in doing so, we must forgive those who harmed us whether we think they deserve it or not. From a secular perspective this seems bizarre, but Christian forgiveness places the focus on Christ and not the perpetrator. It should also be noted that forgiveness does not require reconciliation. That can only be achieved by the perpetrator's confession of their wrongful behavior with a change in behavior that is consistent over time. While forgiveness can be difficult, it can be achieved through fervent prayer with Jesus as the guide. It is required of all Christians. Reconciliation on the other hand is not. Perpetrators must deal with the consequences of their behavior and sometimes reconciliation is not possible.

Dr. Lewis Herman's third stage involves the survivor reconnecting to life in the present. She makes the astute point that the old self has been destroyed by the trauma and in its wake emerges a new self. The old self had beliefs that needed to be challenged and refuted. The new self-rises to a new day with a sustaining faith. Dr. Lewis Herman's use of the phrase sustaining faith resonated with me because it causes me to think about Hebrews 11. The first verse in Chapter 11 of Hebrews (KJV), "Now faith is the substance of things hoped for, the evidence of things not seen." Hebrews Chapter 11 talks about how faith was demonstrated in the Old Testament by Noah, Abraham, Sarah and Jacob. They all demonstrated a measure of faith I had not clearly understood until I began this journey with God's help. Each of them were tasked by God to believe what He had told them before His words became their reality. I had studied God's words in the past. It was only now that His words came alive for me. In Proverbs 3:5-6 (KJV), "Trust in The Lord with all thine heart and lean not unto thine own understanding. In all thy ways acknowledge Him, and He shall direct thy paths." For me to truly appreciate Hebrews 11:1, I had to fully embrace Proverbs 3:5-6. Too much of my life I spent trying to understand the ways of God. This is folly as God says in Isaiah 55:8 (KJV) "For my thoughts are not your thoughts. And your ways are not my ways, saith The Lord."

By meditating on His Word, its truth began to shake the very foundation of my faith. Faith is a full submission to God's will. As a survivor of trauma that is a difficult task. Submission in the beginning is a dirty word. I felt that I submitted to some of the abuse I had experience in my childhood. I consciously agreed that I should submit to God's will, but unconsciously I bristled against it. I began to have a deeper understanding of God's word, and could apply it more in my life. The work of Dr. Lewis Herman also challenged my concept of what true submission was. After all God is not my mother, Gene, or Susan. He is not a man in that He is not capable of harming me. God is love, He loves us more than any human could. He loves me more than I will ever be able to understand.

Once I realized that I can truly submit to His will by faith, just as Noah, Abraham, Sarah and Jacob had, the weight of sorrow and despair lifted off me. Circumstances in my life didn't suddenly change, but my perception of them did. God helped me to focus outward to do his will. I needed to have renewed faith to begin an ongoing conversation with trauma survivors about overcoming the effects of the past. It is interesting that by allowing God to use me, I became connected to today in a way I hadn't since I was a young child in Newark. It appeared that most of my life I wore the albatross of sorrow from my past, but no longer. As I connected to a sense of purpose, I was thrust into today. Each day afforded me a new opportunity to read about the treatment of trauma so I could learn about myself and be prepared to help others. I could learn how to end the relationship I had with trauma.

The end of this relationship with trauma is not sealed with a kiss or a lasting embrace. There is no farewell glance. It is instead like standing in a powerful windstorm; it buffets my soul. I struggle at times to keep my footing. At the moment I think I will lose my balance, it is gone. In its wake is the unoccupied part of my soul. Its emptiness begs to be filled with new memories and experiences. Doubt and insecurity had taken a heavy toll on me. Its heavy weight removed, I am now able to see the clear purpose that the Lord has for my life. Unlike Lot's wife, I will not look back for what the Lord has in store is ahead of me.

A future of human uncertainty that is girded by divine certainty that God is with me. That He orders my steps. As stated in Roman 8:28 (KJV), "As we know all things work together for good to them who love God, to them that are called according to His purpose." That purpose is to be conformed into the image of Christ. As Christ has suffered, I must suffer. Most importantly, as He has triumphed so will I. All things are working for my good if I have focused on the One who has restored my soul by providing my help through His created beings, many of whom may not honor him as their creator, but I see clearly that He is. I trade my relationship with trauma for a renewed relationship with Jesus and I will tell His story of renewal to all who will listen. Praise His Holy Name.

TRANSFORMATION

Something miraculous happened to me when I prayed to Jesus to save me from yet another beating when I was six years old. Jesus entered my life. I wish I could tell you that moment started a love affair with my Savior. After all, He had just saved my bruised little body from a beating I could not have possibly endured. Perhaps I was too young to fully comprehend the magnitude of that moment. Maybe I thought there would be no other beatings. This was not the case. I think those other beatings confused me. As a young child, I felt Jesus was there and could save me from Gene, but it seemed that he was simply watching over me, waiting for me to summon Him again.

Instead of turning to Jesus, I chose to cope in another way. I began another dangerous thought process; I believed in my own goodness. I recognized Gene as evil. I chose to become his opposite. It seemed that the more I despised him, the more self-righteous I felt. This self-righteousness became the seed for future anger. It was this anger that spurred me on after I was kicked out of my family home. I struggled with self-esteem issues as an adult. Anger helped me distracted me from my low self-regard. I never felt like I fit in. I blamed those feelings on Gene and my mother. I thought they should have raised me better. What I couldn't see, or perhaps what I didn't want to see, was that I was also angry at Jesus. He was watching over me, but I thought He didn't intervene. That anger, however, lay dormant in my unconscious. I was not ready to address it.

I now realize how that anger toward God was manifested in the way I related to Him. As a young adult, I would attend church sporadically. I would often blame the pastor, rationalizing my lack of attendance on boring sermons. What is amazing to me is that God placed people in my life that presented His Word to me. Sharon's late father was a deacon at the 48th Street Baptist Church. He would often lead bible study with his family, which now included me. After his death, Sharon took the lead in finding a church for our family. I knew that, as the husband and father, I should have had that responsibility. Back then, I felt I was too busy at work, but I was still mad at God. I knew God's Word but I did not allow it to seep into the recesses of my heart. A pastor at our church encouraged me to read a chapter from the book of Proverbs every day as part of my daily devotion. Since there are thirty-one chapters, I could complete the book each month if I followed his advice. I did that for about three months. I read the words, but did not internalize them.

I floated through life. I was now in the future I had dreamt of as a battered child. I had a loving family. I had more money that I'd ever had before. I had a big house. I had my dream car. I appeared to be successful. I began to deceive myself. I forgot how Jesus had entered my life when I was six years old. It seemed so long ago. I believed in my own success even though at that time I felt empty. I had all that I had wanted, but I still lacked contentment in my life. I looked for pleasure in so many material things. That didn't help. I started to look to people who didn't know me as Burt, but as Dr. Jones. I craved female attention. I knew that it was wrong to curry their favor. I knew what the Bible said about infidelity. I felt justified to act on my desires based on the amount of psychological damage I had endured. I was blind to all to the people I would hurt, Sharon, my children, the people who had respect for me and the women I had relationships with. It was all about me and my search for solace in the arms of women. I now realize just how far I was from God.

God, however, did not give up on me. He started to talk to me through music. While listening to Kirk Franklin and the Family's debut album. I noticed how the words of several of the songs touched me in a way no secular song ever did. When I listened to the album while driving, I would become overcome with sadness. Often I had to pull over and weep uncontrollably. Song after song from various gospel artists would have the same effect on me. Where was all this sadness coming from? I struggled to answer to that question. I listened to more and more gospel music. I now know that it was cathartic for me. The lyrics spoke to bible verses that I was familiar with. The combination of the singing and the music touched my soul. God was allowing me to see how deep was the well of pain and anguish I had inside of me. In my Dr. Jones persona, I thought that my cup was half full. I was now struggling to hold onto that thought. The Lord knew it was not what I truly felt, I was deceiving myself. I was seeking God in gospel music, but God knew I needed to be in the midst of a community that believed in the bible. I had to go back to church.

As I was struggled with my life and its meaning in the face of losing my jobs in the Medicare/Medicaid programs, I was broken. I shuffled around with my head lowered, my shoulders slumped. I remember one of my co-workers, Linda Graham, talking glowingly about her church. She would invite to attend Enon Tabernacle Baptist Church. I remembered how much I enjoyed the CD she had given me. I had thought about visiting her church since I lived in the neighborhood. I was initially reluctant to attend such a big church. I was ashamed to be looked down on by "church people." I viewed "church people" as devout, well dressed, prosperous people. People who would look down on me. After all, I was an adulterer, I had left my family, I had a child out of wedlock and my finances were in shambles. I was embarrassed to be called Dr. Jones because I knew what that title had meant to me but that image was forever shattered. Despite my insecurities, I decided I needed to go. I thought I could hide out in the balcony.

I went to a Saturday evening service at Enon in the fall of 2007. I walked sheepishly into the sanctuary dressed casually. I didn't make eye contact with anyone as I headed to the balcony. I felt like a fish out of water. As I made my way to my seat I was impressed by the music I heard. It was like the gospel music I had been listening to. What I enjoyed the most was the sermon by the Senior Pastor Dr. Alyn E. Waller. I have heard several good sermons in the past and that sermon was one of the best.

There was something unique about Pastor Waller's sermons. I felt that he was talking *about* me. In this sanctuary of more than three thousand people, he was directing his sermon to *me*. His words connected to my soul. God was using Pastor Waller to speak to me. I was overwhelmed by his words. Tears streamed from my eyes, I became even more aware of my brokenness. I am quite sure there are many pastors who are as gifted as Pastor Waller, but I was so glad that God had presented this man of God to me. I continued to attend Enon. I hid in the balcony and wept quietly as I allowed God to heal me.

Those early days at Enon started my journey into truly knowing the Lord. I eventually joined the congregation. I thought that I was doing something for God. I started reading the bible more often, which is not saying much since I hardly read it at all. I was reading the bible with the understanding that I needed to model Christian values.

I soon began to attend Enon on a regular basis. My knowledge of the Holy Bible began to increase. After Susan and I were engaged she attended and eventually joined Enon. At that time, I had been reading the bible more, Susan was much more dedicated to her study that I was. I continued to convince myself that I didn't have the time to read the bible because I had so much work to do. There was still threads of the Dr. Jones persona I was not aware of.

It wasn't until we were separated that I found myself back at the foot of the cross. I was at the end of myself. Suddenly the Dr. Jones persona was not more important than my marriage. After a few weeks, I prayed to God, asking Him to save my marriage. I was asking Him to help Susan with her anger. As I mentioned earlier, God said that she was not the one who was angry, I had the problem with anger. That caused me to weep uncontrollably. I had come face to face with my own truth. That truth was that *I* was leading my life and not God. I had not consulted God when I made any decisions in my life. Past decisions were fueled by anger. I could not deny that anymore. At that time, though, I was aware only of the anger I had against Gene, my mother, and Susan. I now realize that my anger was far deeper than that. I knew I had to look for treatment for my trauma as anger was just one manifestation of it.

I started to research treatment methods for trauma survivors. One treatment that was of interest to me was Eye Movement Desensitization and Reprocessing also known as EMDR, a treatment modality created by psychologist Dr. Francine Shapiro in 1987, which I mentioned earlier. Dr. Shapiro noticed that by calling to mind distressful thoughts, the use of side to side eye movements are useful in producing symptomatic relief. Dr. Shapiro believes that trauma survivors have unprocessed memories and these unprocessed memories cause trauma survivors to behave in ways they find distressing.

What appealed to me the most about Dr. Shapiro's description of EMDR was her statement that her method of therapy was not about blame. I needed to hear that. I had spent most my life blaming Gene, my mother and Susan for how I was feeling. That blame was the fuel for my rage. It was that rage that blinded me from my pain. I could finally find valid answers to the question haunting my life. I have tried many forms of therapy in the past with no success.

I must admit that I was somewhat incredulous at my first appointment. I didn't know what to expect. My therapist performed what I thought was a thorough evaluation of my childhood trauma. No therapist before her seemed to even want to discuss my traumatic past. We spent the first two sessions discussing my childhood trauma and the relationships I had an opportunity to talk frankly about my family of origin. I told my therapist about what I had read about trauma and EMDR.

On our third appointment I had my first set of EMDR. I focused on a long-forgotten memory. My therapist had an EMDR unit that played tones that alternated from my right ear to left ear in synch with small vibration of pods in my left and right hand. The tone in my right ear would match the vibration in my right hand with the same occurring on my left side. After setting up the equipment we began our first session, or set as they are commonly called. The first memory processed was when I was fifteen years old, Gene was supposed pick me up at the old Sears department store located on Roosevelt Boulevard after I had any evening driving school class. I guess it was the less threatening memory. I explained the memory to my therapist while my eyes were closed. It was a cold winter night. I wasn't dressed appropriately for the weather. I figured Gene would be there on time. I figured wrong.

After I had waited about an hour, I began to feel cold. My therapist asked me to concentrate on what I was experiencing while I listened to the tones and felt the vibrations. I felt my eyes moving left to right rapidly. I then had a flashback to that night. I heard the rushing of the traffic as I waited for Gene. I trembled as if responding to the cold even though the temperature in the room was comfortable. I felt as frightened as I had that night. I didn't know if he was coming. I remembered coughing so hard I was nearly nauseous. After walking around the block for about three more hours, thinking, I had forgotten where we were supposed to meet, Gene arrived. There was no apology. I was angry as I got into the car. I listened to the music he was playing on his radio as I shivered on the way home. I was amazed by that first set. I was convinced that EMDR would be helpful for me.

EMDR helps trauma survivors make connections to memories long forgotten by tapping into the unconscious where many memories good and bad hide. I was so used to struggling with many horrible memories, that I rarely tried to remember good ones. One of the memories my therapist wanted me to recall was a memory of a safe place. As we worked on this, I thought of a memory I hadn't I thought of since I was a five-year-old boy. It was a lovely memory of when I was living in Newark. One sunny fall morning, I walked into the kitchen of my friend Robert's apartment. I remember how the bright sun streamed through the blinds in the windows and the smell of freshly made pancakes. Robert's mother's sunny smile seemed to escort me to my plate. Connected to that memory was a feeling of family I have never felt in my life since. In truth, my childhood in Philadelphia did not allow for that experience. I didn't allow myself to experience a sense of family with Sharon or with Susan. Nevertheless, I treasured that memory. I can even still smell those delicious pancakes.

My most memorable EMDR set was when we were working on memories of Newark Burt. In the set, I was transformed back to when I was that happy child. I was walking with my head up, and my shoulders pulled back. I had a sense of confidence I had not experience since then. My heart was filled with such pride. I was overwhelmed as tears of joy streamed down my face as I wore a broad smile. It was truly an amazing experience. I still smile when I think of that set.

One of the effects of EMDR that took be by surprise was that I became painfully aware of how often I had dissociated in the past. Early into my EMDR therapy I became aware of an internal construct, a place I created that I had existed in. There was a part of me that was very critical that kept me on task. It would analyze my every thought and every action. It helped me to perform well academically in elementary school, middle school and high school. It helped me to achieve during my undergraduate studies. It also helped me to avoid focusing on the negative impact Gene was having on my life. I knew I was not like him. To me Gene was pure evil. I started to delude myself into believing in my own basic goodness.

The part of me that I think served me the best was the part I called the fantasizer. It helped me not to focus on the horrors of the day; instead I focused on the future. As a child, one of my first fantasies was to dream about how different my life would be once I became a doctor. I was focused on what my life would change. Gone would be my shabby ill-fitting clothes. I wouldn't go to bed hungry because there would be enough to eat. Instead of living in a cramped house with my siblings, I would live in a huge mansion with more rooms than I needed. I wouldn't have to take public transportation because I would drive a Mercedes Benz or a Jaguar. Since I loved comic books, I imagined having enough comic books to open a store. Even though I had very little material possessions as a child, those dreams gave me a sense of purpose. Those days I had my life and my dreams ahead of me.

Those parts served me well. They gave me a sense of purpose. They prevented me from falling into the grips of alcohol like my father. It was what kept me from venting my rage. I didn't want to be like Gene. I was afraid that if I became angry, I would become like him. He was my only model for how anger was expressed. Perhaps I would hurt someone and end up in prison. I was allowing the part of me that was hurt, Hurt Burt, to avoid the pain of today by focusing on a better future.

As I proceeded with EMDR, I became painfully aware of my own Internal Family System as described by psychologist Richard C. Schwartz, PhD. In Internal Family System or IFS, Dr. Schwartz views consciousness as composed of parts or subpersonalities. Each has its own positive function for the individual. Dr. Schwartz divides those part into managers, exiles and firefighters. Managers are the parts that play a protective role. Managers protect the self from being hurt. Exiles are the parts that are being hurt. They bear the burden of shame, fear and trauma. Firefighters are the parts that present themselves when the exiles demand attention. Firefighters serve to distract the individual from attending to the pain experienced by the exile.

As I viewed myself in terms of the IFS model I saw myself in the following ways. My hypercritical self and fantasizer served to help me manage my emotions. They served to protect the part of me that was hurt, cope with emotional and physical abuse. While the physical wounds that afflicted Hurt Burt would heal, they left emotional wounds that remained as tender today as when they were first created. It is amazing to me how I could avoid experiencing the depth and breadth of my pain. My firefighters were manifested through my overspending. I lavished myself with various material items to soothe myself. It is only now that I can see why those purchases never satisfied me.

I expended a great deal of energy not dealing with my internal pain. As I worked through some of those issues I gradually no longer needed the fantasizer. It appeared that the fantasizer was integral in my dissociations. The fantasizer kept me from facing the pain of my trauma. I noticed that after EMDR sets I would be in a lingering dissociative fog after a set in the initial phase of treatment. I would process these experiences with my therapist. I was losing my old ways of coping with stress. Those ways served to camouflage my dissociative states. I was no longer distracted. Without any cover, I was left in a foggy state. I became aware of how often this happened. This explained why I was so distant from Sharon and the kids. I chose to isolate myself in my bedroom, much like I did as a young child. With this observation, I saw parallels to how I must have felt I when I was drawing in my room on the third floor. I realized that while I was drawing, I was able dissociate and enter the colorful fantasy world of comic books. I drew quite a bit when I was in my adolescent and preteen years, the years when I suffered the most abuse.

Although I still love to draw, I would become frustrated whenever I sat down to draw as an adult. That childlike enthusiasm was not there. The impetus, the driving force for it was gone. There was no threat of emotional or physical abuse. That threat caused me to dissociate and thus drive into the escape of fantasy that fueled my ability to draw. It is only now that I can see the connection. Without the trauma, there is no need to draw. In this journey, I must learn how to uncouple trauma from the joy I received from drawing. I must repurpose this skill purely for my pleasure and not as a way to escape psychological pain.

I also noticed what was happening to me whenever Susan and I had an argument. The emotional tone of her voice triggered feelings I had when Gene would yell at me. As I listened to her I would have an emotional flashback. A tidal wave of fear would engulf me. After that wave washed over me, I would feel frozen in place. At this point, all I could hear was the emotional tone of her words. No matter what she said to me, all I heard was, "You're an idiot, why did you think this would ever work out?" I felt like my body was empty, like I was afloat. At first it would take a few minutes to get myself together. As we argued more often, those feelings would last for hours and even days. I didn't know how to explain this experience to her, and I had no idea what was happening to me at the time. I felt lost.

As time passed, and I prayed and read more about Complex PTSD, I began to understand Susan's purpose in my life. The Lord was demonstrating to me what He knew and what I refused to see through this relationship. I had to stop running away from my trauma. I had to face it. I was so good at avoiding my trauma that I had convinced myself that I had moved past it. I never realized how my anger was a cancer to my soul. It had metastasized in every aspect of my being. I was only able to understand this after I faced the sting of going through my second divorce. My anger had truly blinded me. Anger was the reason I wore a mask that cover my pain.

It was enlightening for me to read about Complex PTSD through the writings of Dr. Judith Lewis Herman, Dr. Francine Shapiro and Dr. Bessel Van der Kolk. It was eye-opening to me. It was amazing for me to read information that I been familiar with but had never applied to myself. I understood how unconscious wishes and desires of past events drove behaviors in others but I was so focused on my conscious awareness of my traumatic past, that I missed the unconscious aspect. I knew it was the reason why I suffered from low self-esteem.

I harbored an unhealthy amount of anger toward Gene and my mother. I superficially applied Christian thought, which was that I needed to forgive them as Christ forgave me. That made sense to me. I prayed about it. I felt that was the right thing to do and I met with both individually and told them I forgave them. I was dismayed though, when I found that over time my anger toward them would resurface. I couldn't figure out why that happened. I now realize that it was because of the unconscious memories of the trauma I had never processed. EMDR gave me an opportunity to process those memories.

Once I started EMDR I was amazed at all the memories that surfaced, many in between sessions with my therapist. I expected that I would have to deal with many bad memories. What I had not planned on was the positive memories of my childhood. I had grown so accustomed to painting my entire childhood with the broad brush of abuse that I had robbed myself of the tender sweet moments I had lived through. I had forgotten the closeness my siblings and I shared as kids who were close in age. And the magic and fantasy I love in comic books. More important, I had forgotten about a tender moment of my childhood. It was a comforting memory I used during EMDR therapy. I had shared many pancake breakfasts with childhood friends in Newark. When I recalled that memory at the age of fifty-four, it brought a broad smile to my face. I hadn't thought about it for decades.

I had once distilled my entire childhood down to events that fueled my anger, which I used to push me to academic success. In that process, I viewed myself as collateral damage to my trauma. I felt damaged by my past. What I lost in the process was that I robbed myself of the happiness due to me because of my success, despite my past. I never appreciated getting my high school diploma, Associates degree, Bachelor of Science degree or Doctorate of Medicine or any other career accolades. I chose to minimize those achievements even though many people would have been ecstatic with them. It wasn't Gene or my mother who robbed me of my sense of accomplishment. I was the one who did that. EMDR helped me to face that reality.

EMDR helped me to psychologically get out of my own way, in a way that no other form of therapy or self-talk could accomplish. I became aware of a lot of emotional turmoil. Unknown to me, bits and pieces of unprocessed memories were wreaking havoc in my subconscious. Some of those memories would surface during EMDR sessions while others would coalesce in between sessions. I felt like EMDR was still operating in my unconscious much like an app running in the background of my smartphone. I felt that I was slowly changing for the better. The funny thing was that I thought I would feel happier. But what happened was that I was feeling more alive.

EMDR helped me for the first time face the fear I'd battled since I was a young child. The fear of an anticipated beating that was always with me, causing an ever-present uneasiness. On the other side of that same coin was the pain of the shame and self-loathing I endured. As a child, I could not endure either situation, but as a healing adult I could face them. As an adult, I could wrap my arms around that fearful child within me and shield him from the torrential rain of shame and self-loathing with my new sense of self-worth. I was developing an inner strength that was dormant since my time as Newark Burt.

Prior to EMDR, I was victim of my past. Every day my unconscious was run ragged by past events. Once I began to process these events, I became more focused in the present. I was not viewing life through the lens of the past anymore. I could now appreciate the light of today. That light is sometimes bright and sometimes dim, but it is not connected to the past. I am living my life in a different way, a more balanced way. The events of my life haven't changed. I still have financial difficulties. I am still going through a divorce with Susan. My relationship with my older children is not the best. What did change was my ability to cope with those issues. I am far more accepting of myself. I can accept that I had made the best decisions I could based on how I viewed the world at that time. I know I still have work to do to resolve these issues. The difference today is that I am not wasting time beating myself up for not making those choices. I realize I did the best I could.

ALLOWING JESUS IN THE ROOM

My greatest transformation came when I allowed Jesus into my heart. Though I had waxed and waned in my relationship with Him, His love for me never wavered. He seemed to speak strongest to me through gospel music. That was always a comfort to me. I knew He could be a comfort to many of the individuals I had the privilege to treat. The idea of talking about religious experience in the practice of psychiatry was frowned upon by many of my supervisors during my training. It was as if the practice of psychiatry was above all religious experiences and to do so was to pander to the equivalent of superstition. It was as if all that could be known about what motivated the human mind could be found in a psychiatric textbook. I knew that there was a lot that could be explained in a textbook, but whatever changed George from a high school bully or helped Aaron overcome drugs wasn't written there, it was in the Bible.

I still struggled with how and when to introduce Jesus Christ to help someone heal from their despair. I knew it should not proselytize to someone in distress, because that was not the expectation of the person I was treating and it could be construed as a way of taking advantage of them. Over time the Lord would speak to my heart as I would evaluate people in emotional distress. I didn't know if it was right to share my faith with people I was evaluating. One day the Lord answered that question for me. It had been my practice during my evaluations that if I noticed the person I was evaluating in emotional turmoil, I would try uplift them in some manner. I mention some of the strengths they had previously identified to me. This was often met with mixed responses. As I became more experienced, I would discuss Christian values to those who professed a Christian faith. In others, I would express Christian themes, though I'd avoid discussing Christianity directly. By doing this I noticed that I could connect with their distress and give them a measure of hope. Despite positive reinforcement on several occasions, I often debated if it was an appropriate thing to do. That all changed after one particular case.

One day, while I was performing a forensic evaluation, I met a defendant whose evaluation challenged my concern about sharing my faith. This job was important for me for several reasons. First, it provided my sole source of income during a dark period in my career, my exclusion from the Medicaid/Medicare program. Second, and in many ways, more importantly, it gave me a sense of purpose. I gave hope to some of the defendants who provided me a window of opportunity to do so. On this day, I evaluated a woman, I'll call her Donna, who had been convicted of third degree murder. I have changed identifying elements of this case to protect her confidentiality, but the key elements of her story remain. The judge presiding over her case determined that perhaps she could benefit from mental health treatment and wanted to take that into consideration during the sentencing phase of her trial.

I noticed as Donna entered the examination room that she was tall and slightly overweight. She was slouched over which made her appear shorter than she was. She was holding her stomach with one hand and held a tissue in her other hand. I could not take my eyes off her as she sat down in front of the clear shatterproof glass that separated us. What drew my attention to her as she entered the room was the fact that she was crying. This was unusual because most of the defendants I evaluated were usually withdrawn, angry or even apathetic. I almost never saw anyone cry because by the time that I evaluated them, months would have passed and they had dealt with their feelings regarding their trial prior to seeing me. Many defendants have reached some resolution one way or the other about their situation. Donna clearly had not. I was not accustomed to such raw emotion. As I performed my evaluation I actively listened for any way I could help beyond the treatment recommendations I would make. Those recommendations would be for treatment months from the time of the evaluation, however; she needed something that day. During our discussion, Donna mentioned that she was a Christian. I was glad to hear that. I silently asked the Lord to help me help His child.

I listened to the story of her life. Donna had been sexually abused by her mother's boyfriend since she was a young child. When she finally told her mother about the abuse when she was a preteen, her mother did not believe her and she was kicked out of the house. Tears streamed down her face as she told me that part of her story. She said she went to work at bar as a teenager. She told me she reached puberty at an early age and appeared older than she truly was. She met a man who treated her well, and eventually married him. They were married for a few years before she found out that he was unfaithful to her when she contracted a venereal disease. Brokenhearted she started using drugs and alcohol to ease her pain. On the day of her arrest, she'd gotten into an argument with a female neighbor while they were both intoxicated. The neighbor pulled out a knife. Donna fought to get the knife away from her. In the ensuing struggle, they both received lacerations. Her neighbor's wounds proved to be fatal. A she told me that she wept loudly. I felt the depth of her sadness. Her despair tested my composure. A tear escaped from one of my eyes and I quickly wiped it away. I quietly prayed to the Lord to please help me find something to tell her.

The Lord laid on my heart the book of Job. I asked Donna if she'd ever heard of the book of Job. She said that she had. I said, then you know that in the book of Job, God allowed the devil to test Job to prove the strength of Job's faith. I told her that Job lost everything in his life much in the same way she had lost everything, her family, her husband and now her freedom. It was then that I noticed she was no longer crying. She was wiping her eyes. A little smile was forming in the corners of her mouth.

I asked if she thought that she could get a copy of the Bible once she got back to the prison where she was being held. She said that she could. Then she said something that truly amazed me. She said that she had brought a part of the Bible with her today. That was what she was holding under her shirt, not her stomach. I figured that it must be some part of the New Testament as many people prefer to read that part since it documents the life of Jesus. I asked what part of the Bible she had. She said she had one part: the book of Job. I repeated to her, "Only the book of Job." She nodded her head, while she wept again. I was shocked. We praised God together and I finished the evaluation. As I left the examination room, I had to go to the adjacent examination room to compose myself as tears fell freely from my face. I received confirmation from the Lord that day that He wanted me to share His Word with all who were willing. What He also let me know was that the sharing of the Word was not just for those I evaluated, it was for me as well.

I continue to look for opportunities to allow Jesus to use me to give comfort to many of the people I evaluate. What we all want, is to be *heard* and not just *listened* to. The people I evaluate want to be sure that I am in the moment with them. So many people complain about interviews with psychiatrists who are so busy documenting the session that there is little to no eye contact. This creates an emotional distance for some, which causes them to emotionally withdraw or shutdown.

It is said that the eyes are the windows to the soul. It is important for me to make eye contact with the person I am evaluating. By making eye contact I demonstrate that I see the person in front of me, that I am aware of them physically and emotionally. In maintaining eye contact I can notice nonverbal communications: the pause when responding to a question, the avoidance of eye contact, and facial expressions that contradict their words. I have had the honor of evaluating so many trauma survivors, of hearing about their experiences. Many do so while in emotional turmoil. I listen actively to gather information where they show tremendous strength or compassion. Once they are finished telling me their story, I reflect their story back to them. Just being willing to listen can be helpful, but providing a measure of hope is far more powerful.

If the person telling the story is a Christian, reciting passages in the Bible gives them an additional comfort that I can only explain as the presence of the Holy Spirit. I thank God for allowing me to witness this on so many cases. To see someone who entered the office, their spirit broken, shoulders slouched, and a deep pain in their eyes transformed after sharing their experience and have the privilege to apply biblical stories to their experience can be transformative. To then see them walk out standing straighter and even being able to smile is truly a blessing to behold.

I began my journey into wellness, obsessed with researching all the available information on Complex PTSD. I discovered in this process that I learned best by listening to audiobooks. I was amazed that as I listened, I could make connections to past life events. One of the first books I listened to was Dr. Judith Lewis Herman's *Trauma and Recovery*. It was transformative. Dr. Lewis Herman's excellent treatise on how psychiatry has viewed the treatment of trauma throughout history discusses how Dr. Sigmund Freud, the founder of psychoanalysis, discovered the root cause for hysteria. Hysteria had become a pejorative term to describe behavior in women that men did not understand.

Dr. Freud initially discovered that many of the women, who were of a lower social economic class, had been sexually abused. He published his early findings based on eighteen case studies in 1896 in the article "The Aetiology of Hysteria." A year later he started to back away from his findings because of the high prevalence of hysteria in all social strata, including the bourgeois families for whom he had established his practice in Vienna. His theory was not politically palatable. He later restated his theory of hysteria to make it more acceptable. It is out of this experience, he developed his theory of psychoanalysis, where allegations of sexual abuse were considered metaphors representing life struggles. In the beginning, he listened to women who shared their horrors with him but based on social pressure, he stopped listening to them. I was intrigued by the notion that someone of Dr. Freud's status in the history of psychiatry would bow to social pressure to deny the pain that his patients had endured.

Dr. Lewis Herman documents in her book how the treatment of trauma survivors has never been the priority of modern psychiatry because many of those seeking treatment were women. After World War I, many men returning home were noted too have what was called combat neurosis. Many of them suffered from feelings of helplessness and fear after the war. These men often screamed and wept uncontrollably just like women who were called hysterical. Initially, British psychologist Charles Myers who evaluated some of the early cases, attributed it to the concussive effects of exploding shells. He said the men suffered from shell shock.

There were two periods in history that impacted the need for treatment for trauma survivors. Both events were based on political movements in the 1970s. One of those events was the aftermath of the Vietnam War on many who struggled to cope with the horrors that they had faced during this violent time. Many of these veterans also returned home to face a country that did not honor them for fighting in an unpopular war. The antiwar sentiment along with the "national experience of a discredited war" added to the burden of the psychological trauma they faced. Many Vietnam War veterans sought support outside of the Veteran's Administration because they felt their voices were not being heard. These veterans formed support groups with other veterans to discuss their common experiences.

The other event was the Feminist movement. During that time many women suffered in silence. Their battlefield was in their homes and on their jobs. In a mental healthcare field dominated by male treatment providers, their feelings were minimized. Since they could not find a voice within the community of treatment providers, they used their own and created a movement in which their voices could not be silenced. Dr. Lewis Herman so eloquently discussed how the treatment of trauma survivors were made by political movements that forced psychiatry to recognize their need for clinical attention. In 1980, the American Psychiatry Association's diagnostic manual added Post Traumatic Stress Disorder as a diagnosis that requires treatment.

Dr. Lewis Herman has been an advocate for the recognition of the full spectrum of conditions that trauma survivors cope with. In 1992, she published an article in *The Journal of Traumatic Stress* titled "Complex PTSD: A Syndrome in Survivors of Prolonged and Repeated Trauma." In that article, Dr. Lewis Herman discusses trauma that occurs in a chronic fashion in prisons, concentration camps, slave labor camps and even in family homes. In reading the article, I understood how my childhood trauma had a lingering effect on me. Even though there were many horrific events throughout my childhood, the chronic nature of it caused me to psychologically adapt. Dr. Lewis Herman says that repetitive trauma causes survivors to become hypervigilant, anxious and agitated without any baseline state of calm or comfort. Dr. Lewis Herman has petitioned to no avail to have Complex PTSD added to *The American Psychiatry Association's Diagnostic Statistical Manual.*

Psychologist Peter Walker in his book, *Complex PTSD: From Surviving to Thriving*, talks about the concept of emotional flashbacks. Emotional flashbacks are feeling states where survivors relive the worst emotional times of their childhood. Everything feels overwhelming and confusing to them. It is an intense response to emotional memories. I now realize that I had been experiencing these emotional flashbacks for years. I knew that during arguments with Susan, I would feel overwhelmed and frozen. At the end, I would be emotionally numb. I didn't initially understand what was happening to me. As I look back over my life, I realize I've had many of those episodes. Those past events were not triggered by an argument, but by stressful events such as being kicked out of my childhood home or losing my job and being placed on the exclusion list for Medicare/Medicaid providers. I sought treatment with therapists who did not recognize that I was suffering from Complex PTSD and my past treatment was not successful.

I researched what my treatment options were. I wanted to have an open mind to what types of treatment were available. I was not interested in dogma. As part of my medical training I was aware that authorities in a given field often present their information as the only answer. I wanted to avoid that type of thinking. I recognize that there is truth in everything, but that ultimate truth rests in God not man. For example, in the instances of intractable cases of peptic ulcer disease, the treatment was a surgical procedure, Billroth I and Billroth II as an elective treatment option in the 1960s. These procedures required that part of the damaged stomach be removed. In the 1970s it was determined that peptic disease was due to stimulation of histamine receptors. Peptic ulcer disease was then treated by the drug Tagamet, which caused a decrease in the need for the Bilroth procedures.

Eventually treatment of peptic ulcer disease shifted to a class of medications called proton pump inhibitors which caused a decreased in stomach acid which was later thought to damage the stomach lining. Gastroenterologist Dr. Courtney Houchen, Chief of digestive diseases at the Oklahoma University Medical Center, states that a commonly held belief at the time was that peptic ulcers were caused by excessive acid, thus the phrase "no acid, no ulcer" was commonly used by Gastroenterologists. By the 1990s it was determined that the bacteria Helicobacter Pylori was the cause of many peptic ulcers. Many people were then treated with antibiotics. I'm sure that patients who had elective Billroth procedures could have been treated with antibiotics for Helicobacter Pylori but the science at that time did not support that. Perhaps some time in the future, treatment for peptic ulcer disease may change to something else. The truth is, God knows the ultimate truth and man is forever in search for it.

The reason why I discuss the issue of Helicobacter Pylori is to stress the importance of keeping up to date with the latest treatment modalities for PTSD. I would also resist anyone who presents a treatment option in a dogmatic fashion. Although many will present their information as the answer for PTSD, remember only God knows the truth. Man's knowledge of truth is based on the best science of the time. Also remember that the scientific community is slow to embrace anything new. In my review of the treatment options for PTSD, I was amazed by the variety of methods used to treat it.

In Dr. Bessel Van der Kolk's book *The Body Keeps the Score*, a variety of treatment options are discussed. While I was aware of EMDR and neurofeedback, I was impressed by his discussion of what I thought were alternative forms of care that I was not aware of, such as yoga, massage therapy and theater.

One therapy modality I find potentially interesting in the treatment of trauma survivors is hip-hop therapy. I've had several conversations with my friend and colleague Ronald Crawford who is the author of *Who is the Best Rapper? Biggie, Jay-Z or Nas*. In his book, he discusses the roots of hip-hop music and how it has been incorporated into therapy by many other therapists. Mr. Crawford processes the lyrics of many rap artists by discussing their meaning to the people he treats in his group sessions; many of them are trauma survivors. He uses the music in an intriguing way by engaging them in the therapeutic process by speaking a language they understand.

FEAR

During my journey, I came face to face with my greatest enemy: fear. Fear grabbed hold of the core of my being and would not let go. It held my joy hostage. Whenever things were going well for me it would show up and fill me with doubt. It kept me vigilant and on edge. It was my psychological albatross. In the past I thought that I could contain it, overcome it by sheer will, by the power of positive thinking. This adversary was far too cunning, far too complex to be disposed of by mere positive thought. I thought that I understood what my fear was, that it had to do with being rejected. Or perhaps it had something to do with my fear of people finding out that I was a trauma survivor.

I worried that they would realize that the great childhood they imagined I had was not real, and that I was broken in ways like the people I treated. I thought I would be treated differently. This was not the case when I started to share my traumatic past with others. I was surprised with how receptive people were. In fact, by sharing my experience I began a dialogue with other survivors of trauma. I decided that it wasn't the fear of people discovering my traumatic past, it was the fear of fear itself. Dr. Van der Kolk described this phenomenon and how it manifests in *The Body Keeps the Score*.

Dr. Van der Kolk writes that individuals who are exposed to trauma learn over time to feel unsafe within their own bodies. The past nibbles away at their conscious awareness of body sensations. As their bodies are bombarded with physical warning signs, they ignore them. They ignore their own intuitions and exist in a numbing awareness of their environment. They become emotionally detached and hide from themselves.

As time passed, I became slowly and painfully aware of how fear had taken residence within my body. Fear had found a safe haven in every organ and in all my cells. Before I began this journey, I thought that I had conquered the fear of my past. It was only after engaging in specific treatment that I realized I was still holding onto fear. Treatment allowed me to become aware of the impact my childhood trauma had on my behavior. In many ways, this fear had been running in my unconscious. Every now and then it would percolate into my consciousness. I never looked at those events as being connected. Instead I looked at them as separate. I can now see their connection because as I became aware of my level of fear, I noticed how it affected my body. I tried to overlook my fear but its presence could not be ignored.

I became aware of the impact fear has had on my life as I made progress in therapy. I thought facing the demons of my past would free me from their icy grasp. But I was only peeling back layers of fear. As I peeled away one layer, I had to face another. At its very core was the fear itself. That was the very essence of the damage my trauma had inflicted on my psyche. The unpredictable randomness of my abuse left me in a constant state of readiness. I was hypervigilant all the time. This hypervigilance was at a cost. I had to prepare myself for what was an inevitable episode of horror: Gene's gathering of the children. This would lead to his questions that were delivered in a pejorative fashion. I would stand motionless during his inquisition. I was frozen in place. It was during those times I was immersed in the icy waters of fear. Waves upon waves of anguish would buffet me. I knew the beating with the extension cord was sure to come and it did. I was forever on guard for when Gene would return home. Was he angry? If he was, would this lead to the dreadful whistle and then a vicious beating?

I was always conscious of the subtle nuances of every sound in my childhood home as things could always change. This robbed me of the ability to relax even during calm times. I felt the quiet times were simply a prelude. Surely panic and chaos were just around the corner. This vigilance had a devastating effect on me as I constantly maintained a state of readiness. Consciously, I thought I could relax, but the truth of the matter was I'd lost that ability years ago. When Dr. Van Der Kolk writes that the body keeps the score he is so right. My body, remembered and kept this state of readiness. I was always tense and uptight.

As a child, I loved to play basketball with my brothers and the kids in the neighborhood. I was average. Okay less than average, but I enjoyed playing the game nonetheless. There were times, however, when the older more talented kids would watch and cheer us all on. I noticed that when they would encourage me, I'd freeze up. Suddenly, I would miss shots I could easily make. As all eyes were on me I would lose the coordination I needed to perform. As I look back, I see that I viewed their attention, any attention, as a sign that I needed to be ready. I needed to stand at attention and survey my surroundings. I was stuck in a paradox. I wanted to play basketball and stand at attention at the same time. My body manifested this conflict as an errant shot that would lead to laughter that fueled embarrassment and magnified my fear.

There was another way I noticed how fear had taken over my body. As a young child, I loved drawing comic book characters. This was inspired by my love for the brightly colored comic books of my youth. Whenever I drew I became engrossed in the fantasy world of superheroes. In doing so, I was drawn away from the chaotic world of my youth. I was able to suppress my fear and hone my drawing skills. As I moved from childhood to adulthood, I wanted to rekindle my love for drawing so I purchased art supplies.

I can look back at any situation where attention was paid to me and realize that it made me nervous. It didn't matter if that attention was positive. I viewed it as a confrontation and I desperately avoided all confrontation. I was incredibly adept at it, that is until I married Susan. Before we started dating, we sometime had disagreements that I viewed as confrontational. This would cause me to distance myself from her. We'd eventually sort things out and our relationship blossomed. This worked out well for us until we married. When we had our disagreements, I would retreat inward. She wanted me to respond to her questions, but I was frozen in a state of hypervigilance. I would have an emotional flashback, although I didn't know that at the time. It felt like Gene was lining me up to be berated and beaten.

Through therapy I learned that I had become so skilled at avoiding confrontation that I failed to realize what was driving it. It was the fear of a beating, and my avoidance of experiencing the fear itself. Fear, which is a natural emotion that requires a fight or flight response in humans. It soon became something that I wanted to avoid at all costs. This, however, is not practical because fear is part of the human experience. I didn't have to be afraid of fear. I needed to relearn its usefulness in my life. Before I could do that, I had to realize how I had learned to distort its role in my life.

Fear had also driven me to a form of blindness. It prevented me from seeing myself as I was. I'd always had a fear of being alone. I thought it was because I needed to be around people. I believed their affection would soothe my shattered psyche. What I realized was that even around them, I still felt alone. Try as I might I could not escape this fact. God in His infinite wisdom allowed me through my free will to create a set of circumstances in which I ended up living alone. Away from my children. Separated from my second wife. Alone. Alone to cry over the aches of the past.

At this point I started praying fervently, more than I had never prayed in my life. Many days and nights I prayed to God to relieve me of my pain. There were also many days I would weep in joy for the tender mercies He bestowed upon me. Over time I realize that my fear had caused me to focus on the external world. To look for signs of calamity and danger that just weren't there. By being alone I had to face the fear and the knowledge of the extent of my brokenness. It hurt to know the full of the extent that this brokenness had on my life. But God showed me that I was not afraid of being alone because I needed people. What I really needed was to know myself first.

I also was waiting for some future time when I would be happy and I had my life together. A time where I would have a smile on my face and spout bible verses to all who would listen. That is not what God wanted. What He wanted was a relationship with Him. He knew me before I was born. He knew all the mistakes I would made and will make. Even with that knowledge, He still loves me. Despite my educational background, it took me fifty-five years to understand what God already knew. I *am* worthy. He has a love for me that I could never fully understand. I, in my fleshly nature, can only understand human love. God's love is so much more. He allows me to learn from my missteps and lovingly guides me along the right path. He also revealed to me that my fear of being alone also involved my fear of being in His presence. I am now beginning to fully appreciate His love for me and to realize what He always wanted for me. That is to simply accept His love.

I had to place my head in the mouth of the lion of fear I had created. I willingly did it because I knew that as God protected Daniel in the lion's den, He would protect me. He allowed me to face my fears and live to tell of His Glory. It was soon apparent to me how pervasive my fear had become when I understood that it was throughout my body. I was quivering with fear physically and emotionally. It was clear that besides EMDR, I needed self-care on three levels: the surface of my body, the inner workings of my body, and the core of my body.

In taking care of the surface of my body, it was important to have monthly massages. Massage therapy helps to release tension in tight muscle of the extremities, the back, and the neck. Emotional energy had tightened my muscles. Regular massages helped loosen and align them so that they could function properly. My posture improved and I walked with more confidence. Physical exercise such as weight lifting and running on my treadmill were also helpful.

To take care of the inner workings of the body and the mind, I started my practice of yoga. When I went to my first class, I realized that I had a misconception of what yoga was. I thought it involved some light movements and chanting, I thought it would be quite easy. What I found out was it was quite strenuous and there was not as much chanting as I'd thought. The focus was on the breath. I found it to be quite invigorating and I looked forward to attending weekly sessions.

Since I found out that yoga was not about chanting, I decided to pursue Transcendental Meditation(TM). I recently went to an introductory meeting at the Philadelphia Transcendental Meditation Center in Jenkintown, PA. I found out that training was conducted over four consecutive days and the next course I could attend would be given a month later. I was excited and looked forward to my training. When I started the course, I was told that Transcendental Meditation is not a religious experience; it is based on the Vedic tradition. The Vedic tradition is noted for shaping Hinduism. I was given a mantra, which I was told was a meaningless word. Although I did feel some benefit from Transcendental Meditation, the idea that I was repeating a mantra whose meaning I didn't know bothered me.

I began my TM course with some doubt. I was looking forward to discovering how it would help me cope with this new chapter in my life. In the workshop I was told that TM works independent of whether the practitioner believes in it or not. That was reminiscent of what I read about EMDR. I took comfort in that. After beginning my TM course, I wondered if I was meditating correctly. My instructor assured me that I was performing my meditation as expected. I noticed after my first few attempts at meditation I felt relaxed.

The effectiveness of TM was put to the test after a few days into my practice. I was invited to a retirement luncheon for a dear colleague, Christine Abdur-Rahim. She had served Gaudenzia, Inc. for thirty-two years. She was a tireless servant for women in need of mental health and substance abuse treatment. She had always been supportive of me at Gaudenzia. There was no way I would miss her luncheon. There was just one issue: the luncheon was being held at the Hilton Hotel on City Avenue. That was where Susan and I had our wedding reception and I worried about having an emotional flashback. I decided that I would still go. There were several banquet rooms and I decided that it was unlikely the luncheon it would be held in the same room. Well God arranged for it to be in the very same room where we held our reception. I was surprised that I was not triggered by it. I didn't have an emotional flashback. I did feel sad, but that sadness was not overwhelming. I was surprised. If I had not started the meditation process, I don't know if I would have enjoyed myself at the luncheon as much as I did. I knew then that meditation was working for me.

As I practiced TM, I noticed that issues I had been praying about would enter my mind often as I focused on my mantra. I soon found my mind shifting to prayer. In this form of meditation I was receiving the similar benefits I received with TM in a practice that supported my Christian faith. This lead me to pursue knowledge on Christian meditation. I revised my meditation practice and researched Christian meditation. I reviewed Thomas Merton's book *Contemplative Prayer* and James Finley's book, *Meditation for Christians: Entering the Mind of Christ*. In listening to both audiobooks, I learned the importance of focusing on bible verses as well as attributes of God while meditating.

As I meditated, I felt God's presence in a way that was different from my daily prayers. It was far more intimate. I became committed to this practice. It helps to quiet my mind so that I can hear God better because I'm not distracted by random thoughts. Christian meditation requires discipline to focus on developing the right relationship with God. That relationship consists of my singular focus on His Glory and His Majesty as well as His Love for me. I felt more connected to Him. Bible study, prayer and meditation became my daily means of worship.

ATLANTA

Life can be difficult at times. I found myself in that space while I was deep into writing this book. I became weary of the struggle to stay focused on it. I had been so busy working that I would ignore how tired I was. I hadn't taken a vacation for two years, not since 2014 when Susan and I went to Las Vegas to celebrate our third anniversary. That vacation was a horrible experience for me because we had an argument that forced me to hide out in the bathroom. I suffered what I came to later understand was an emotional flashback. That experience left an enduring mark on my psyche.

I decided to book a trip to Atlanta, Georgia in August of 2016. I had talked to several colleagues about their previous vacations to Atlanta. They all seemed to enjoy themselves. I decided to see if I would agree with their assessment. I had put off taking a vacation because I felt that I was too busy at work to do so. I had initially convinced myself that I didn't need one. One of the benefits of the work I had completed in this journey was that I learned to be honest with myself. My work would still be waiting for me when I got back. I was mentally worn down by the monotony of my work schedule. I think part of my reluctance to go on a vacation was that I had to go alone. That was a new experience for me but I didn't need the distraction of another person. This would be another opportunity for me to learn more about myself.

As I waited for my flight to Atlanta I was struck by the fact that this would be my first flight alone. The reality of it gave me pause. In the past I might have started an internal monologue that would have viewed this trip through the prism of a failed life. There was no family to travel with me, Susan was not an option. I was not in a relationship, so there was no woman in my life to invite. I decided to view this trip through the lens of reality. I needed rest and relaxation in a different venue. This was a new chapter in my life, and I wasn't alone; God was with me. I left my fatigued spirit in Philadelphia at 3:05 PM as my plane took flight.

I arrived safely in at Hartsfield-Jackson Atlanta International Airport at 4:40 PM. I was excited to start my vacation. After changing my clothes in my hotel suite at the Ritz-Carlton on Peachtree Street, I went to Sweet Georgia's Juke Joint and had a sumptuous meal while I listened to a Rhythm and Blues band. What a great way to start my vacation. Once I returned to my room, I had a restless night. I tossed and turned. I was thinking about that trip to Las Vegas. I eventually went to sleep only to be awaked at 12:52

AM. The first thing on my mind was the revelation that I had discovered the root cause of my anger.

I thought back to when I was six years old and I prayed to Jesus. I remembered how I had romanticized that pivotal event in my life. There was a part of that experience I could not face then but was ready to deal with now. It had to do with a lie had told myself. That lie was that I would never become angry because I didn't want to be like Gene. The truth of the matter was I was angry all the time and it wasn't at Gene; it was at God. It took me many years to face this truth. The boy that was physically and emotionally abused prayed to God for relief from a situation he didn't think he deserved. As I look back on that situation, I couldn't acknowledge my anger because to do so would mean I would have to look at the depth of despair associated with my life. I wanted to hold on to the few shreds of the free-spirited child of Newark who still lived in my heart. The cup had to be half full. There was no point in looking at the dark dismal half empty cup. It served no purpose for me then.

Today I can look back at that time and see that I was angry at God because He allowed me to be brutalized. I guess in a way I thought that I was not worthy of expressing my anger. Just as my ancestors during slavery, I had learned that to express my anger would only lead to more pain. And who would listen? I learned it was pointless to resist the main perpetrator, Gene. At the moment, I prayed for God to enter my life, which He did, but I decided to keep Him at a distance. I didn't know how to deal with a God who could stop one beating, but didn't stop others. I buried this anger deep into my unconscious. I couldn't understand as a young child how God was working things out for my good.

I always suffered from some form of depression. It never stopped me from achieving my goals, but it did rob me of fully enjoying them. Various forms of talk therapy and brief trials of antidepressant medications didn't seem to help. Sigmund Freud's paper, "Mourning and Melancholia," suggests that depression is anger turned inward, which made sense to me. I was making myself sick by not expressing my anger. I couldn't express my anger because I didn't know its root cause.

As time passed I would demonstrate my anger toward God by purposely disobeying His Word. I would have affairs, and spend my finances on material possessions, out of a sense of pride. This pride was a cover for my anger. The Bible states in Proverbs 16:18

(NIV), pride comes before the fall, and fall I did. In the process, I hurt my five children, my stepdaughter, ex-wife and my soon to be ex-wife. My life was a chaotic storm. In times such as these I reflected on Kirk Franklin's introductory song on his *Songs in the Storm* album. As an adult that song helped me to understand what the scriptures were saying to me. Paul talked about our sinful nature in Romans 7:18-20 (NIV). "For I know that good itself does not dwell in me, that is, in my sinful nature. For I have the desire to do what is good, but I cannot carry it out. For I do not the good I want to do, but the evil I do not want to do—this I keep doing. Now if I do what I do not want to do, it is no longer I who do it, but it is sin living in me that does it."

As I began to accept that my unresolved anger had played a role in my past behavior, I was appreciative of how EMDR was able to bring this issue to my consciousness during this moment of emotional clarity. I had to acknowledge that while that level of anger had existed in the past, it was not driving me in the present because I was aware of how God was with me every step of my journey.

It is in this season of my life that I can truly look back and see God's hand in my life. By man's standards, I would be the last person giving anyone advice on how to live their life or how to overcome their struggles. But my journey was never about me, the purpose was never about me it is about Him who sent me. It is He who could use someone like me to show the way to the person who can provide the ultimate hope. Jesus.

I was feeling refreshed when I returned home a few days later. My trip to Atlanta was invigorating. I went to check my mail on August 24, three days after my return. I saw two large brown envelopes among the usual junk mail and bills. They were from a law office. One had been delivered on August 16th and the other August 20th. I opened the first one carefully, wondering what it was. It was notification that Susan had filed for a divorce. The second envelope was a copy of what was in the first one. A sense of relief washed over me, after all, we'd been separated for over two years, and in Pennsylvania, that met legal criteria for a divorce. I understood that Susan could not wait any longer for me to figure my life out. She obviously did not want her life to be held in limbo. She had every right to file for divorce. I felt that this phase in my life was over. Then suddenly the finality of my thoughts struck me and I fell into a deep pit of despair.

I'd been praying for God's will regarding our marriage. I knew that God could intervene and change our hearts and bring us closer. He also could allow us to drift apart if it was at least the will of one of us. It was Susan's will. God does not force us to go against our will. His desire is that we align our will with His, but in His permissive will He allows us to follow our own. I guess I thought that God would follow my heart's desire and that we would be reconciled once I was at the end of this journey I was on. I felt that I was close, but not close enough for Susan.

Rather than become mad at her, I became mad at God, just like the hurt child from my past. This wasn't supposed to happen. Even though I knew it was a possibility, the reality devastated me. I spent the next few days in a whirlwind of despair. I was barely able to function. I drifted through the day. Once I got home I would think about the end of my marriage and I would curl up in a ball a cry inconsolably for ten to fifteen minutes, two to three times a night. I would cry from the pit of my soul. I was in dire emotional pain.

After a few days, I wondered why I was crying so much. If I looked at the tumultuous nature of our marriage, this result should not be surprising. I prayed for God to make a way out of no way, but the truth of the matter was that Susan and I had barely spoke about our marriage for more than a year. We would have infrequent, superficial conversations. It wasn't like we were working toward a reconciliation. I wondered what was the root cause of my soul stirring. I had a similar experience when first listened to gospel music. Back then I'd wonder where all this emotion was coming from. As I prayed to God for understanding, He helped me see a connection that I could not see before.

I had never grieved for the horror of my childhood. Sure, after each beating I would cry from the pain of the beating, but not for the emotional turmoil. Those feelings I suppressed. I only had access to them during periods of profound distress. Gospel music put me in touch with that distress. Painful life stressors would lift the lid of the emotional teapot where my pain was boiling. I needed the lid to blow off and allow me to feel the full impact of that pain. The thought of the divorce process blew the top off the teapot and I was able for the first time to feel that pain. I guess this was the time for it to happen. God knew that I was prepared for it. Hurt Burt could fully express himself. As much as it hurt, I was better for it. It was cathartic.

JOSEPH

As I consider my life's journey I can't help but think about Joseph. Genesis, Chapter 37, begins to document his story. He was the youngest and favorite son of Israel. As a child, when Joseph told his older brothers about a dream he had, they became furious because in that dream he told them that he would eventually rule over them. Infuriated by this dream his brothers plotted against him and sold him into slavery. Joseph was sold to Potiphar who was one of the Pharaoh's officials. The Lord was with Joseph and he prospered while he lived with Potiphar. Potiphar placed a great deal of trust in Joseph and left him in charge of his household. Potiphar was only concerned about the food he ate. He entrusted everything else to Joseph.

Joseph was a handsome man and drew the attention of Potiphar's wife. She wanted to have an affair with him. He refused her advances as he did not want to betray Potiphar's trust. One day Potiphar's wife attended to her duties and had arranged for all the servants to leave the house before Joseph arrived. When he arrived, she grabbed his cloak and again asked Joseph to come to bed with her. He ran out of the house while she held his cloak in her hands. Holding his cloak, she ran to the servants and told them that Joseph had attempted to rape her, but she screamed and Joseph ran away. She told Potiphar this story, he became furious and had Joseph imprisoned.

While in prison the Lord was with him. The Lord granted Joseph favor with the prison warden. Joseph was put in charge of the prisoners. The warden paid no attention to those under Joseph's care. While in prison Joseph met two of Pharaoh's officials, the cupbearer and the baker. They both had unsettling dreams but didn't know what they meant. Joseph told them that dream interpretations belong to God. They told Joseph their dreams and the Lord used Joseph to interpret them. He told the cupbearer that in three days he would be restored back to his position. He asked the cupbearer to remember him when he was in the Pharaoh's presence. Joseph also interpreted the dream of the baker. He told the baker that in three days the Pharaoh would cut off his head and impale him on a pole. These events occurred just as Joseph said. While in the presence of the Pharaoh, the cupbearer did not remember Joseph.

Genesis 41 states that two years later the Pharaoh had a dream that disturbed him. When he had a second disturbing dream, he asked all the magicians and wise men of Egypt to interpret them. They could not. It was at that time the cupbearer remembered Joseph. The cupbearer told Pharaoh how Joseph correctly interpreted his dream. The Pharaoh sent for Joseph and asked him to interpret his dreams. Joseph told him that he could not, but God could. He asked the Pharaoh to tell him his dreams so that through him, God could interpret them. The Pharaoh did and Joseph said that God revealed to him that his dreams foretold of a seven-year period of famine and that Egypt would need to store up food to survive it. The Pharaoh was pleased with Joseph and soon placed him in charge of Egypt. The famine did come as God had told Joseph, and Egypt was prepared. Egypt had storehouses of food and sold some to others throughout the world.

Genesis 42 documents how the famine would eventually affect Joseph's father Jacob. As he was old, he sent Joseph's brothers to Egypt to buy food so they would not die. His brothers took the long trek to Egypt at their father's request. Joseph recognized his brothers as they approached, but they did not recognize him. Joseph asked them about their father and found out he had a younger brother. Joseph requested that they bring their younger brother to him in Egypt. Jacob was reluctant to send his youngest son Benjamin, because he thought he had already lost Joseph and didn't want to lose Benjamin as well. His other sons told Jacob that they promised to bring Benjamin before Joseph. Eventually, Benjamin was sent as told in Genesis 43.

Joseph eventually revealed himself to his brothers who were immediately overcome with fear because they knew what they had done to him. Since Joseph was a powerful man in Egypt, they felt that they surely would be punished. Joseph, being the man of God he was, showered them with love and then said the words that resonates with my soul in Genesis 50:20 (KJV) "But as for you, ye thought evil against me; but God meant it unto good, to bring pass, as it is this day, to save much people alive."

Joseph's story beautifully illustrates the meaning of forgiveness. If I am honest I have struggled with the concept of forgiveness in its true sense. I used to think that forgiveness was a magnanimous gesture I extended to Gene and my mother for what had happened in my childhood. It was my gift to them. It was so good of me to do that. That was not forgiveness at all, because unconsciously I wanted them to apologize and spend the rest of their lives making it up to me. When that didn't occur, I became angry all over again. I realized that I had not forgiven them at all. Then I came to understand that forgiveness wasn't for them, it was for me. I had to learn what forgiveness meant, not from a secular sense but from the Christian perspective.

I was only focused on myself as the injured party. What was undergirding that position was my basic belief of my own goodness. I totally ignored the Word of God, which says in Romans 3:23 (KJV) "All have sinned and come short of the Glory of God." I became so invested in what had been done to me that I became ignorant of my own sin. In Matthew 7:3-5 (NIV), "Why do you look at the speck of sawdust in your brother's eye and pay no attention to the plank in your own eye. How can you say to your brother, 'Let me take the speck out of your eye' when all the time there is a plank in your own eye? You hypocrite, first take the plank out of your own eye, and then you will see clearly to remove the speck from your brother's eye."

It is so amazing how you can read scripture and not get its deeper meaning until the Lord allows life's events to illustrate its truth. Those verses lead me to a truer understanding of what forgiveness truly is. For so long, I felt so justified in my anger toward Gene and my mother that I was blind by to plank of anger in the eye of my soul. It was that anger that caused me to develop an unhealthy narcissism that placed my needs above others. I didn't care who I hurt because I was convinced that I had a right to be happy. That plank in my eye blinded me to the hurt I inflicted on my first wife and children when I left. The hurt inflicted on the women I had affairs with. It even led me to realize how I hurt myself when I had to deal with the emotional aftermath of these decisions. How dare I allow this anger to consume me like a raging fire? I had to remove this plank from the eye of my soul.

I found myself living in an apartment all alone. Broken and battered by all the bad decisions I made in my life. I was at the foot of the cross. My heart was aching in way it had never ached before. I was at the darkest abyss of despair. That was when I found that I was not alone. That's when I found out that Jesus was with me. He was always with me. I chose not to acknowledge Him. I thought with all my education I could figure this thing out. I was wrong. I cried to Him and He heard my cry. I remember the joy I felt when I finally surrendered to Him. Jesus showered me with His love. That was Jesus' sweet gift to me. I now understood that I did not deserve it, but He still gave it to me. I smile when I think of that.

He showed me how I could remove that plank from my eye. He let me know that I had to give up on my pursuit of happiness and focus on the gift He had given me. That gift is the ability listen to those under my care while I wait for the opportunity to talk about Him. He required that I be obedient to His will. I found that when I was obedient, I felt better about the situations in my life. I knew it was not up to me, it was up to Him. He slowly gave me the strength to make changes in my life. I was now able to do things that I could never do before. He was acting through me. He showed me how to avoid using anger to cover my vulnerabilities. Instead I found renewed strength in those vulnerabilities.

What was most helpful to me was when I finally learned to trust in God. I was once angry and bitter towards God. I now realize that my anger was based on my feeble attempts to understand the ways of God. I looked at my child abuse, financial collapse, marital and parental struggles as a series of negative events that should not have happened. I was misguided in that kind of thinking. Isaiah 55:8 (NIV) states, "For my thoughts are not your thoughts, neither are your ways my ways," declares the Lord." What I had to understand was that I had no right to be angry at God in the first place. I needed to trust Him. Just like Joseph did. All the events of my life served to shape me into the person I am today. I have learned far more about myself during the difficult times in my life that the happier ones. In the difficult times, I would cry out to the Lord. Each time He heard my cry. Each time, he made a way out of no way. Each event I viewed as negative would stretch me and mold me into a better version of myself.

I am reminded of Jerry Bridges' book, *Trusting God*. In this book, he gives an excellent illustration of how trials contribute to spiritual growth. "One of the many fascinating events in the emergence of the Cecropia moth from its cocoon—an event that occurs only with much struggle on the part of the moth to free itself. The story is frequently told of someone who watched a moth go through its struggle—the viewer snipped the shell of the cocoon. Soon the moth came out with its wings all crimped and shriveled. But as the person watched, the wings remained weak. The moth, which in a few moments would have stretched those wings to fly, was now doomed to crawling out its brief life in the frustration of never being the beautiful creature God created it to be.

What the person did not realize was that the struggle to emerge from the cocoon was an essential part of developing the muscle system of the moth's body and pushing body fluids out into the wings to expand them. By cutting short the moth's struggle, the watcher had actually crippled the moth and doomed its existence."

Jerry Bridges uses this description to illustrate how God uses trials to strengthen us. James 1:3 (NIV), "because you know that the testing of your faith produces perseverance." Truly indeed, my trials did cause me to endure a great deal of stress, which caused me to call out to God. The emotional agony I endured caused me to tap into internal resources God knew I had. Through all that I have endured, I am now closer to God than I ever was. I have learned to trust God. He has seen me through everything. He has given me a sense of peace. I have developed spiritual muscles that will help me to cope with trials that I may have to endure in the future.

The material things of the world I coveted in the past did not have the same luster. I felt best when I was serving Him. He in turn guided my steps to various books to read. I began to have conversation with people and He used those conversations to nourish my soul. I began to have compassion for Gene and my mother. It is still a process. God is still working with me but I now understand that until I extend full forgiveness to them, I cannot expect full forgiveness for myself.

Matthew 6:12 (KJV) "And forgive us of our debts, as we also have forgiven our debtors." Once I understood the full meaning of that verse, I knew that for me to be in the position to accept forgiveness from others, I had to first extend it to Gene and my mother. What I then realized was how I had depended on my hatred for my existence. It served me well as a young child. It helped me to cope with a horrible situation. But that was in the past, it wasn't now.

I knew that consciously; the problem was unconsciously I didn't. This is how I believe that God used EMDR to help me deal with my unconscious thoughts to bring them in line with my conscious thought. My unconscious was still fueling a world of fantasy that I needed as a child. The hope that Gene and my mother would be people they never were. I am now in the position to accept the fact that they are who they are and to accept them as that. I needed to remove the plank from my eye entirely. Once I did that I could see the speck in their eyes. I could see their need for compassion.

I forgave Gene. On many occasions, he told us of how he was brutally beaten by his own mother. He also told us that he was hard on us to keep us from dropping out of school or using drugs. He never showed us compassion because perhaps no one showed it to him. I thought that I avoided being angry so I wouldn't demonstrate anger the way that he had. Instead, my anger oozed out of my unconscious and manifested in self-destructive behaviors.

I still believe his actions toward us were abominable, but he still needed forgiveness. I, on the other hand had to take responsibility for how I expressed my anger. I cannot blame Gene for that. For many years, I allowed my anger for Gene to drive me. It was the fuel for a part of my success. It also was the fuel for my downfall. That anger was the proverbial chip on my shoulder. It became a major driving force in my life. It fed my low self-esteem. It fed my lack of confidence. It fed my feeling of perpetual misery. I had been coping with misery for so long, I didn't know how life would be without it. It was through EMDR that I can connect to my feelings as Newark Burt. I knew I could survive without the anger because I had lived without anger before I carried its burden.

I forgave my mother. In many ways, it was harder to forgive her than it was to forgive Gene. When I first met Gene, I found him to be a likable guy. He, however was not my father and I loved my father. I never loved Gene. My mother on the other hand was someone I truly loved. I watched how she struggled to study to become a nurse with an unsupportive partner and five small children. I will always admire her persistence and focus through it all. As I mentioned earlier, she was my inspiration to go to medical school.

I faced the ultimate betrayal in my life when she asked me to leave our family home. She told me that Gene wanted me to leave. When I asked Gene why he wanted me to leave and he said it was my mother's idea, I refused to believe that because I considered Gene a liar. However, as time passed I began to see the truth that my tender heart didn't want to see. Gene may have wanted me to leave, but so did my mother. As I recall all the beatings that I sustained at the hands of Gene, several of them for things I didn't do, she never spoke up for me. The woman who I believed was so intelligent hardly ever acknowledged my academic achievements. In the one moment in my life that she could have advocated for me, she didn't.

The betrayal cut me deep. I struggled to fully trust the women in my life after that experience. EMDR allowed me to see how that once special relationship had morphed into a frosty ambivalent one. That twinkle in my eye I had for her was snuffed out. I now realize that my mother was a battered woman, first by my father and then Gene. I see parallels in how she raised us in how I raised my children. Although my children were never physically abused, they did have to deal with an emotionally distant father who, when home, would retreat to his bedroom to watch movies and not connect with them. I retreated to a room and was uninvolved in their lives just like my mother.

Like my mother, I used humor to interact with them. I used humor to mask the self-loathing I lived with. My mother used humor in the same way, I suspect. She loved me the best way she knew how; it just fell short of what I wanted. I strove to find someone to fill the void of love I felt in my life. I tried to do so in many relationships to no avail. Pastor Waller often talks about all of us having a God shaped void that only He can fill. Through this process, I have learned that I need to seek God's love for me. The only way I can truly embrace it is to forgive my mother. Mommy, I forgive you.

I forgive you Susan. From the first time, I met you I noticed that there was something special about you, but I couldn't quite figure it out. At first I thought it was simply your beauty, but that is too easy. I thought it was the way you would confront me on my behavior. No one had ever done that. Gene would comment on my behavior when I was a young child, but as time went by I learned how to hide it from him. I could never do that with you. You had the uncanny ability to peel away the layers of my defenses and you would wound me by touching the tender core of my being.

You could get me to see my hurt self. Once we were married, you stripped away all of my defenses. That made me very angry, to the point I separated from you. In the initial phase of our separation, Jesus revealed to me just how angry I had always been. I then thought I could figure out what I needed to do to restore our marriage. When my plans didn't work, I became more frustrated. I focused my frustration on you. *Why won't you change,* I wondered. The Lord revealed to me that I was the one who needed to change. As I gained more insight into my behavior and unconscious motivations through EMDR, I saw that God was using the stress of our marriage to allow me to see what I had not been aware of for years. I often became bewildered during our arguments. I realize now that I was having emotional flashbacks. I would often become angry with you when they occurred and that was the main reason I avoided arguments. I was suffering from Complex PTSD and was impairing my ability to relate to you in manner that was supportive of you.

After finding out I suffered from Complex PTSD, things began to fall into place for me. I better understood myself. It lead me on this journey to seek out information about Complex PTSD. It gave me a sense of purpose. I need to communicate this information to others. I knew that I wasn't the only person who felt this way. I see now how God has used you to help me find my purpose. So even though we have had many arguments that left me balled up in emotional distress, Susan, I forgive you, and more importantly, I thank you. Our struggles propelled me toward my healing. I only wish that I could have come to that conclusion earlier, but alas it was not God's plan for it to happen until now.

The person I struggled the most to forgive is myself. This is because in a bizarre way I feel like I have let myself down. I also carried a belief from my childhood into adulthood that was detrimental to me: my basic belief in my own goodness. There was a need to hold onto that belief as a young child to distinguish my behavior from Gene's brutality. I conducted myself in ways that I thought were good. I followed all the household rules and I behaved at home. I excelled in school. I performed odd jobs as a kid to earn money to buy clothes so that my mother and Gene wouldn't have to buy them for me. I never was suspended at school. I didn't have a problem with drugs or alcohol. I was never arrested. My behavior however, reinforce my belief that I was good. I learned from my father's death how I would be different from him and demonstrate my love for my future kids. I felt rightfully angry at my mother and Gene when I was asked to leave home. After all I was a good kid.

Now, as an adult, I am reminded of Jesus' words in Mark 10:18 (NIV) "Why do you call me good?" Jesus answered. "No one is good—except God alone." Also in Roman 3:23 (NIV) "For all have sinned and come short of the glory of God." I read those words as a young man, but their deeper meaning came as a challenge to my idea of my own goodness. I fell under the spell of secular goodness. But as God spoke to me through His Word, I became painfully aware of how I fell short of His standard. It wasn't the secular society that set the standard for me, it was, and still is Jesus Christ.

When I tried to compare myself to Him, I saw my many flaws. I looked at my motives. Proverbs 16:2 (NIV), "All a person's ways seem pure to them, but motives are weighed by the Lord." Once I took a realistic view of my motives, I saw a hurt person who had a pattern of using people to fill a bottomless void of validation they could never fill. On the surface, I thought I was doing the right things, but in the end, I realized I had done far more harm than good.

Although I read God's Word, I did not follow His Word when making decisions and God allowed me to see myself in those decisions. God used therapy to help me see the error in my way of thinking. As a hurt person, I could not see it. As I slowly rose from my pain I saw the error of my ways. The greatest error that I committed was that I did not trust God to help me. He was always there waiting for me to ask. He knew I was too hurt to see Him, so He created a way to see Him so much better. I love Him for that.

As much as I struggle to forgive myself for how I have used people in my life, such as the women I have had affairs with. I must forgive myself for how I brought those issues to my first wife Sharon. She deserved better from me. I now see how my struggle with my abusive past created a desire to thirst for adulation from her. She could not slake that thirst, no one could. I left my marriage unaware of the heavy emotional burden I still carried. I brought that into my second marriage with Susan. I now see that I would have been better served by working through those issues. I, however, must keep everything in context. It was in the often-tumultuous relationship with Susan that God thrust me to the end of myself. I had exhausted all the alleged "goodness" in me.

God placed a mirror in front of me. When I looked in the mirror in the past, I would often see remnants of a tortured soul. The mirror God placed in front of me showed me my true self. It was more than just my physical appearance. He showed the appearance of my very soul. I saw my wretchedness. I saw all the evil machinations during my childhood as well as during my adulthood. The mirror also showed the spiritual chasm between me and God. I also saw that He was waiting for me as the father in the parable of the prodigal son. He was waiting for me at the road where I had departed from Him. God used my relationship with Susan to bring me back to Him at the foot of the cross.

I forgive myself for how emotionally withdrawn I was from my beautiful and wonderful children. I never wanted them to be burdened by my childhood. I never even talked to them about my abuse. I highlighted the good things from my childhood, though they were few. I apologize to them for not being more emotionally involved in their lives. I celebrated birthdays, Christmases, and family trips. I told them jokes and funny stories. But I robbed them of seeing their father happy, truly happy with life, not putting on a show for them. I was physically there, but I was dissociating much of the time because those events unconsciously triggered bad memories for me.

I was stuck in an emotional conundrum. On one hand, I wanted to give them a childhood different from mine, but I didn't have the emotional context to enjoy those moments with them. It was like I mechanically performed my duty as a father. I always wore a mask to cover my tortured soul. Sharon was far more actively engaged in their lives and I thank God for that. I thought the best thing I knew how to do was work and make money to buy them things. I worked long hours and they always understood. What my children needed was a more emotionally engaged father.

I foolishly thought that when I separated from Sharon, it would not have much of an effect on them. I was wrong; they were devastated. Even though I hurt them in a profound way, whenever we would spend time together I noticed they had learned to wear a mask just like me. Just like mine, their mask had tortured eyes that betrayed their frozen smile. The separation took a toll on them with behavioral problems in school and poor grades soon followed. I tried to encourage them to talk about their feelings with me not realizing that I had never talked to them about how to express their feeling in the past. They were not willing to talk to the person they felt was destroying the family.

Eventually Sharon and I divorced and I felt an emotional chasm between my children and me. As I became more aware of that emotional distance, it took a toll on me. I questioned myself as a father. I felt responsible for the pain that I caused them. I also saw parallels between my role as their father and the effect my own parents had on me. I was just like them. Like my father, I was self-absorbed in living my life my own way and had not factored my kids into it. Like my mother, an abuse survivor, I was emotionally withdrawn from my kids. Fortunately, I was not emotionally and physically abusive like Gene. But I took no solace in that. I had behaved in a way like both my father and mother. In that manner, I hurt them as I was hurt by my parents. My children deserve better from their father. I struggled with the burden of that knowledge.

God, in His infinite wisdom, allowed me to atone for what I did not pour into my older children by turning what was once a seemingly scandalous event into an opportunity for redemption. My youngest child Camronn was born outside of my marriage to Sharon. We were separated at the time of his birth. I was forty-four years old when he was born, and struggling with shame and guilt at the time of his birth. I had a rocky relationship with his mother. Despite all of this, I did not want to abandon him. I wanted to honor my responsibilities as his father.

My relationship with Camronn's mother soured, but we were able to share custody of him. Although, I would receive some help from Sharon and the older children on the weekends I had him, I functioned as single man, though I was technically separated until I later divorced Sharon. I had shared in the early care of my other children, but never to the extent I did with Camronn. It was a bit bewildering being a father again. I could push through moments of fatigue as I was juggling work and becoming a father for the fifth time.

I now realized that God used the circumstances of Camronn's birth to show me His love in a profound way. Camronn is a free spirit. He has a smile that lights up a room. As a toddler, he had the ability to connect to people with his engaging smile. Once when he was two years old, I took him and my other children to Disneyworld. While we were waiting in a long line for an attraction, he walked to the other families in line and entertained them with smiles and hugs.

They were appreciative of his affection. One family asked if they could take a picture of him. I proudly gave them permission and Camronn flashed his million-dollar smile while he posed for pictures.

When Camronn was in kindergarten, his teacher noticed that he was struggling with his schoolwork. He was tested and it was discovered that he had a developmental disability. He managed to maintain his smile although he struggled with his schoolwork early on. He eventually received the educational support that he needed and has shown good progress. What I noticed early on with him was that he had a passionate desire to please me in anything that he did. It would upset him if he could not complete a homework assignment because he thought he was letting me down. I made sure that he always knew that I loved him and I wanted him to simply do his best.

Camronn, like all my children, is a gift from God. God has allowed me to provide for him consciously what I did not do for my older children. I was truly present with him. The amazing thing was that he was present with me as well. Camronn has the gift of emotional intelligence. I often worry about different issues in my life regarding work, finances and relationships. One day as I was getting Camronn ready for bed, he looked at me and asked, "Daddy, are you okay?" I tried to brush him off saying that I was alright. He moved closer to me, his worried eyes scanned my face and he gave me a look of disbelief. His eyes saw what my words betrayed. At that moment, I felt that this child was concerned about his father in a profound way. Even today at ten years old he amazes me with his emotional intuition. When we are at home together, he will spontaneously say to me, "Daddy I love you." He also will stop playing with his toys or playing with his iPad and walk over and give me a hug. Surprisingly, this usually occurs at times when I needed one.

On Father's Day in 2016, Camronn had a surprise for me. He'd been working with my daughters on a karaoke version of Charlie Puth's song, "One Call Away." He sang the song with nervous passion. He wanted to do his very best, and he did. One line in the song touched me as I watched him sway to the beat. He sang, "Superman got nothing on me, I'm only one call away." He looked at me as he sang from his heart. When he finished, he became overwhelmed with emotion and began to cry as he reached out to me and gave me a tight hug. I thank God for that moment. I appreciate how He uses Camronn to show me the sweet innocent love of my youngest child.

When I look at Camronn, I often see Newark Burt. He reminds of how happy and free-spirited I was as a young child. I had a zest for life. I had the same passion for people as Camronn does. I see myself in him and it makes me smile from deep within every time I think about it. God, through Camronn, has shown me that he can take my life's circumstances and help me to find victory in them.

Most important of all, I forgive myself for how I treated God. The author and finisher of my faith deserved more from me. He was waiting for me at the road where I departed from Him. I turned back to Him, broken and embarrassed with my head bowed as tears streamed from my eyes. I was not worthy to be in His presence. I felt that I had squandered all my riches and all my talents. I felt I had nothing to offer Him. I sobbed as I approached Him in prayer. I screamed aloud, begging Him to forgive me. I trembled in His presence when I was alone with Him praying at the foot of the bed in my apartment. I was never so vulnerable in my life.

In the abyss of my despair, Jesus caressed my head with His hand as He sweetly and gently kissed my forehead. He then nudged me on my chin, looked into my eyes and told me He loved me. *Me.* He told me that He had a plan for me. At that moment, I felt love in a way that I had never experienced before. It wasn't the love I had seen in a Hollywood movie and longed for in my life. It was the love my God always had for me. The person who knew all my faults, all my thoughts, all my motivations and all my brokenness and accepted them. He loved me as I was. He would use my experiences for His Glory. He then wrapped me in the robe of compassion. He placed the ring of my truth on my finger and fed me from the fatted calf of His love.

I saw for the first time what I knew intellectually but now knew experientially, which is that God is love. I must forgive myself for not honoring Him as God. I now realize that. He has removed the scales from my eyes and I see the world in a different way. I fully accept my shortcomings for they prove to me without the shadow of a doubt that there is no goodness in me that is inherently mine. Any goodness that I have is from Jesus. It is in Jesus that I can go on even though my life circumstances have not changed.

I see God's hand in my life. All my life experiences are important. I perceived many of them as bad and some as good. The reality is that they are all important because they represent the many tests I have endured in my life, all of which make up my testimony. I knew in Christ's eyes I was already forgiven, in the past I foolishly refused to accept it. God's love for us is so amazing, we simply have to ask Him for forgiveness and He will forgive us. I asked Him and He forgave me. I must now forgive myself for thinking I was not worthy of it, because I am.

After accepting God's full forgiveness, I had to wrestle with my greatest adversary. It wasn't the devil. No, it was something far more insidious. It was my inability to love myself. In the past, I thought loving myself was a selfish act. I instead I chose to demonstrate selfless love. I was always careful to be sensitive to the needs of others. I would go out of my way to please other people. Funny thing is, I never felt fulfilled. That's because I was looking for fulfillment in human relationships, the only person who fully and completely loves me is Jesus Christ. When I look to Jesus I see the embodiment of Love. In His love, I am filled to the point of overflowing.

Understanding the Journey

Faith

This journey in my life has been a test of my faith. I had to face the veneer of faith I had previously existed in. I had far more confidence in my own abilities than in God. I was enamored by my ability to navigate relationships and conceal my feelings of inferiority. As I became successful in my academic achievements, I minimized those feelings. There were a few occasions when I thanked God, but not as much as I should have. As I look back, I am amazed that I could have any achievements in the face of how little I valued myself. I would view life events as series of good and bad events. I would always look over my shoulders when things were going well waiting for something bad to happen. In my despair, I was unable to see God.

Hebrews 11:1(KJV), "Now faith is the substance of things hoped for, the evidence of things not seen." In the midst of my misery, my faith was challenged. I was so distraught from the aftermath of childhood abuse that I suppressed many of my feelings. I was not conscious to the extent of how it had eroded my faith. It was no wonder that my church attendance was so poor in the past. But today as I let go and let God, I can see His Hand in my life daily. As I look back I am now aware of how He has walked with me despite my failure to acknowledge Him.

I now realize that I must fully submit to Him. Psalm 143:10 (KJV), "Teach me to do Your will. You are my God; Let Your good

Spirit lead me on level ground." I need to turn away from my abilities and focus on what God has in store for me. I admit that it can be frightening, but that is because I am viewing my situation from a human perspective. Fortunately, God has greater plans for me than I could ever imagine. I only need to trust in Him.

Hope

As I look toward my future, I sometimes have moments of apprehension. I must admit that I even have some measure of fear. How will this book be received? Will it reach the people I want to help? Have I done all I can in the telling of my story? I reflected on this as I drove to work one blistering hot summer day. I stopped at my favorite Sunoco gas station on Mount Airy Avenue in Philadelphia. My gas tank was nearly empty, so I decided to fill it up as much as possible with thirty dollars. As I pulled up to the pump, I saw a thin teenager sitting on a rail next to the pump. When I got out of the car he introduced himself. His name was Kaseem, and he asked me in a pleasant voice if he could pump my gas. He reminded me of myself when I was his age. I figured I would help him out and give him five dollars for his service.

I felt the oppressive heat as I watched Kaseem pump the gas. What made matters worse was the gas pump was incredibly slow. I could see that the young man was confused. He tried to shake the hose to make the pump work faster as he nervously looked at me. I smiled at him and told it was okay even though I was uncomfortable as I waited outside my car. What would usually take about a few minutes was taking almost fifteen. In that time though I saw something that took my breath away. Kaseem asked every motorist for an opportunity to pump their gas. Many would barely look at him while they said no. One lady said no, but only did so because he was working with my slow pump. I told him to go ahead and pump her gas so that he could earn another tip. What was remarkable about him was even though many motorists declined his offer, he thanked them. Once those motorists finished pumping their own gas, he would tell them to have a blessed day as they drove away. His demeanor was so admirable that several motorists who'd pumped their own gas gave him a tip anyway.

In Kaseem, I saw myself as that young child in Newark, full of youthful confidence. I also saw a young man who must be dealing with some form of adversity. There had to be a reason he was panhandling at a gas station. As a young man, I was never able to exude the confidence he had. I know I could not have handled so many repeated rejections with his aplomb. Kaseem lifted my mood. I told him how he had touched me by the way he conducted himself. I told him that God is using him and encouraged him to continue to serve Him. I decided to give him a twenty-dollar tip. He was shocked. I told him he deserved it.

I remember Joshua 10:25 (NIV), "… Do not be afraid; do not be discouraged. Be strong and courageous. This is what the Lord will do to all the enemies you are going to fight." As I drove away, I was overcome by that experience. I wept as I thought of how God had given me that moment when I needed it. He had given me the courage to fight through my insecurities. I had been so consumed by own pain and my insecurities that I forgot what God's purpose for me is. It is to serve others. As I was bathed in that experience, I felt that God knew I needed it. In that moment, the Lord told me that I had to pivot away from myself and to focus on my audience—

childhood abuse survivors, and the people who care for and love them. I should remain vulnerable in order that the Lord's work in me can be clearly visible. It is not about me, but about Him who sent me. I needed to put my trust in God and I needed to remain full of hope.

Love

As a child, I had family members show affection to me, but it was divided. I was one of six children. We all received affection equally, but no one ever told me that they loved me as an individual. The closest I came to that was the brief time we lived with my maternal grandparents while my mother was in Philadelphia. They showed more affection than other family members. The interesting thing was that since they were both deaf and mute, they could show me that they loved me, but they could never say the words "I love you." I never heard anyone say that they loved me until I was nineteen, when I was dating Sharon. When she told me that she loved me, I replied, "Why did you say that?" I simply didn't know how to respond to those words.

I had always struggled with low self-esteem. The years of physical and emotional abuse took its heaviest toll on my ability to accept love. That inability to accept love caused me to have a distorted view of love. I recognized that I had a void in my life. I knew that I was not raised in a loving home. I wanted to find the love I missed. Oddly enough, I thought by watching family shows like T*he Brady Bunch* in the 1970s, I would understand what a loving family looked like. I wished that Mike Brady was my father. He was patient and loving with his kids. I wanted that for myself. I especially enjoyed watching *The Courtship of Eddie's Father*. I admired little Eddie, because he had a father that loved him so much. He paid careful attention to Eddie. It was in watching those shows that I reluctantly had to accept the truth that I did not have that kind of love in my home.

As I grew into an adult, I never fully understood the impact that the images of love on television and in the movies impacted my life. The love shown on television shows and in movies was far too simplistic. Love has always been depicted as a positive emotion. The sun shone brightly on those who were in love. There was no end to the smiles on their faces. This was not my experience. I spent my life in search of finding that kind of love. I search for this love in people and in material things. The newness of relationships and the possession of new items was always intoxicating to me. That feeling however did not last and I would end up disappointed. I would reflect on what I thought was my failure and redouble my efforts. Time and time again I would end up disappointed.

I then discovered Kamal Ravikant's book, *Love Yourself Like Your Life Depends on It*. In it Mr. Ravikant stresses the importance of learning to love yourself. This was eye-opening for me. I thought the idea of self-love was far too narcissistic for me. I struggled with how to reconcile that concept with my Christian faith. I then thought of what Jesus said in Matthew 12:30-31(NIV), "Love the Lord your God with all your heart and with all your soul and with all your strength. The second is this: 'Love your neighbor as yourself.' There is no commandment greater than these." I read verse 31 with new eyes. No wonder I was never fulfilled by the love I received from others, I could not fully accept that love. I struggled to accept their love because I did not think I was worthy of it. I would in turn gave a form of love that was self-serving. I was hoping that their love would fulfill me because I struggled to love myself.

Mr. Ravikant talks about the importance of loving yourself to the point where you are overflowing with love. I understood that I was sharing love from a deficit. This made the love I gave a selfish kind of love. I was giving love with the idea I would be getting something in return. The problem with that way of thinking, was that no one could fill me up with love because I was not able to adequately receive it. Jesus' words struck me when I realized that I couldn't truly love others because I didn't love myself. It wasn't the responsibility of others to help me to understand love because I had the ability to do that myself. My inability to love myself also showed me how I was also limiting myself. I thought I needed others to have confidence in me when in truth I was ignoring the fact that I had no confidence in myself.

My awareness of this issue affected my view of the world. I now realize I have been holding myself back. I look over the tapestry of my life and weep in joy knowing the real reason I went through all the heartache and pain. It wasn't to tell my story. It was telling His story, God's story. As I look back over my life, I can see now what I could not see then. God was molding me and shaping me. At times these processes hurt, and the problems in my life seemed impossible to bear. But just as pressure applied to coal produces a diamond and fire applied to gold refines it, God's Hand molded me into the person I am today. I am not perfect, but He who is within me is . I am perfected through Him. I thank God for my childhood. I thank God for my adulthood. I thank God for the valleys in my life. I met Him in those valleys. He was there at the mountain tops but I was too busy praising myself to see Him. In the valley, I couldn't help but see His Glory and Majesty.

I thank my ancestors who endured horrors I can never imagine. I thank my mother and Gene for shaping me during my formative years. Their lack of genuine affection for me stirred within me a desire to be different to the hurt people to whom I have the honor to provide care for. I developed an understanding of how it felt to be ignored and marginalized by people who were responsible for caring for me. Whenever I saw people who were hurting, my heart reached out to them. I wanted to give them a measure of comfort and compassion. I thank my siblings who put up with my foolishness as we triumphed over our collective past.

I want to apologize to my first wife and my children for not being fully present in their lives. I thought I was, but I now know that I wasn't. I weep as I write this truth. To my second wife, I truly want to thank you. Words cannot express the debt I owe you. God placed you in my life so I could face a truth I was running from. The truth is this: I was broken and only God could restore me. When you talk to me, you speak to my very soul. Your words strip away the flesh of my defense mechanisms and speak to the core of my vulnerability. God has used you to help me face my truth. I was angry with my life, and underneath that anger I was hurt. Because God used you, I was set on this journey. Thank you.

On many days and nights, I cried because I thought I was having a nervous breakdown, I now know what was really happening. It felt like I was losing my mind. I now know that what I was losing was the emotional baggage of my past. I was so used to carrying it that when it was gone I was left with the despair it didn't allow me to see. It was a deep pit of despair. In the valley of my despair, I met someone. Someone who is kind. Someone who understands. Someone who still loved me despite all the mistakes and missteps I made. Someone who loves me. Jesus. He wrapped

His arms around me in that abyss. He looked me in my eyes. He told me that He loves me and could use me. Even me. I then began this journey. It led me to reading His Word in a more committed fashion, to read books and to pray. It lead me to different forms of therapy and more praying. For all that, I thank God. I thank God for you, my readers, for reading this book.

In this journey, I finally found out what I was running from. I was stalked throughout my late childhood by something that pursued me at every turn. I tried to rationalize it away. I tried to understand it. At times, I tried to reason with it, but to no avail. It could not and would not bargain with me, so I chose to try to act like it didn't exist. Yet when I looked over my shoulder, I saw it lurking in the shadows. I tried to outrun it but it kept pace with me. I had to turn around and face my enemy: fear. I once thought I had a fear of being alone, of being rejected, of being a failure. I had to realize that I was so accustomed to feeling fear that I realized that I was afraid of fear itself. A childhood rife with abuse and neglect left me in a state of constant fear. I looked for things and people to rescue me. It never dawned on me that I could rescue myself with God's help. His Word says that in 2 Timothy 1:7 (KJV), "God hath not given us the spirit of fear; but of power, and of love, and of a sound mind."

At times that childhood fear, the fear of waiting in line for my turn to be beaten, or waiting for something to happen that would lead to another beating, lay dormant in my soul. It was the reason I always had a feeling of uneasiness even in calm situations. It was why I was always vigilant. It was why I could never trust my environment. A metaphoric beating was always around the corner. What I have come to understand is that the true basis of my fear was that I no longer wanted to feel as vulnerable as when I was a young child. I did not want to fall victim to a crazed world where the innocent would be punished. A world where physical pain would coexist with emotional turmoil. It was a world there was no one to protect me. I would tremble alone with no hope of rescue. Whenever I was involved in any conflict my mind would wander to that dark place.

My help came in reflecting in the worlds of the bible. Just as in Daniel Chapter 3, when Shadrach, Meshach, and Abednego were thrown into the fiery furnace, which was seven times hotter than normal, King Nebuchadnezzar thought they would be afraid. Instead their faith in God grew stronger. So, strong that they had no fear. Amid the fire that was supposed to consume them, King Nebuchadnezzar saw a fourth person walking around unbound with them. God was with them. In the end, the three men emerged unscathed. It is in this season of my life that I can understood a passage I have read many times before. In the fiery furnace of my own vulnerability, I looked around at the environment for my Comforter. He was there to provide comfort then, just as He does now. I chose to place my faith in Him and not submit to fear.

In this season of my life, I look to the bible to understand the definition of love. 1 Corinthians 13:4-7(NIV), "Love is patient, love is kind. It does not envy. It does not boast; it is not proud. It does not dishonor others, it is not self-seeking, it is not angered, it keeps no records of wrongs. Love does not delight in evil but rejoices with truth." I struggled to fully understand this passage. I needed to focus on how Jesus Christ demonstrates His love for us. In the past I had thought that love was simply an emotion. I was heavily influenced by secular society. Love was never discussed or demonstrated in my childhood home. I had to take my cues from other sources. I carefully watched how love was depicted on television and in movies. But it is so much more.

Love in its truest sense requires action. To be sure there were people in my life that showed acts of love to me. Unfortunately, in the aftermath of trauma, I often focused more attention on the times when they didn't show love in a way I thought I needed it. While I was hurting, I was desperate for human affection, contact, and validation. In this season, I now look at Jesus for the true definition of love. John 15:13 (NIV), "Greater love has no one than this: to lay down one's life for one's friends". Roman 5:8 (NIV), "But God demonstrated His own love for us in this: While we were all sinners, Christ died for us."

This whole experience has given me a purpose. That purpose is to help other abuse survivors know that God has a plan for you. Everything in this world was created by Him. John 1:3 (KJV), "All things were made by Him; and without Him was not anything made that was made." That means that psychotherapy, psychotherapeutic techniques, yoga, theater, massage, exercise, support groups and medications. Even caregivers or group members whether they are a Christian or not, were created by God. Even if the people involved as your support system are not Christians, God still created them. It is also important to attend a supportive church. It is important to be in fellowship with fellow believers. As the bible says in Matthew 18:20, "When two or three are gathered in my name, there I am with them."

Blame

To survivors of childhood abuse it is so easy to feel justified in blaming those individuals who abused us. After all, it was those dreaded individuals who have tortured us so and caused our lives to be what seemed to be damaged beyond repair. While it is true that the individuals are solely responsible for their actions, we are responsible for how we respond to their actions. It is hard to keep from blaming them for our struggles in our lives, but we must so we can heal.

I blamed Gene and my mother for my tortured soul. I blamed them for my feelings of low self-esteem. I wanted to blame them for my periods of depression. They were responsible for my social ineptness. I wanted to heap upon them all of my troubles. What I was oblivious to was how this blame was fueling my anger. In the beginning, I used that anger constructively, to focus on my studies. I channeled that rage to become successful academically. The unfortunate thing is that after I graduated from medical school, my anger did not subside. It grew in intensity. It metastasized to my soul. It became the driving force for several rash decisions I made. At times when I was emotionally hurt, it reared its ugly head. Instead of allowing me to feel hurt, it allowed me to feel pure anger. That anger blinded and kept me from appropriately addressing those issues.

By releasing Gene and my mother from blame, I could free myself to work on my anger.

FINAL THOUGHTS

In *I'm Alright*, I share my journey from childhood innocence to childhood pain, and then to adult victory. It would be a misrepresentation to imply in any way, that this process proceeded in a straight line. Far from it, it has been a long and winding journey and I felt at times like Israel wandering around in the wilderness. I spent more than forty years of my life wandering in my own wilderness, and it was of my own creation. I am reminded of the familiar story of the man caught in a terrible storm. He was a faithful Christian. He heard that the storm threatened to cause the riverbanks to overflow and flood the nearby homes. He was ordered to evacuate his home immediately by town officials. He proudly stated, "I will trust God, and if I am in danger, then God will send a divine miracle to save me."

His neighbors came by his house and said to him, "There is room in our car for you, please come with us!" He said, "No thanks, God will save me." The floodwaters rose higher and approached his steps. A man in canoe paddled by and called to him, "Hurry and come into my canoe, the waters are rising quickly!" But the man again said, "No thanks, God will save me." The floodwater rushed into his house and he had to retreat to his second floor. A police motorboat saw him in a window. "We will come up and rescue you!" the police shouted to him. But again, the man shouted, "No thanks, use your time to save someone else! I have faith that God will save me!"

The floodwaters eventually forced the man to climb onto his roof. A helicopter saw him and dropped a rope ladder. A rescue officer came down the ladder and pleaded with the man, "Grab my hand and I will pull you up!" The man continued to refuse help, stating, "No, thank you! God will save me!" Shortly after that, the rooftop collapsed and the man was carried away by the floodwaters and he drowned.

When in Heaven, the man stood before God and asked, "I put all my faith in You. Why didn't You come and save me?" God replied, "Son, I sent you a warning. I sent you a car. I sent you a canoe. I sent you a motorboat. I sent you a helicopter. What more were you looking for?"

As I look back over the events of my life, I can see how God was providing for me. He was there to answer my prayer as a six-year old child. As a child and as an adult, I thought God would save me in a way I would understand. He had other plans. His ways are not my ways; His thoughts are not my thoughts. He was there in line as I was beaten as a child. He gave me courage to press on after I was asked to leave my childhood home as a young adult. His heart yearned for me to return into relationship with Him when I succumbed to my own lusts. As I struggled to understand my diagnosis of Complex-PTSD, He guided my steps so that I could be more enlightened. At times, I asked Him why I had to suffer so. His reply was like the story above, "What more are you looking for?" He was there every step of the way; I was blinded by my lack of faith.

We know that God created the world and everything and everyone in it. He is the source of all truth. My mistake was in thinking I could figure out the solution to the problems in my life without Him. Like the man in the story, I was blind to the many ways God had offered help to me. I wanted God to help me *my* way not His. I now understand the error in that way of thinking. I pray that you will not make the same mistake. I only ask that you seek the Lord's guidance in your life through fervent prayer and fasting. He will lead you to your solution. If He presents to you psychotherapeutic treatments such as EMDR, Prolonged Exposure, Christian Meditation, among others, be open to them. He may suggest yoga, dance, or music as therapy, utilize them. If He suggests that you diet and exercise, listen to Him. There may be a newly discovered treatment modality that will prove to be helpful. Be open to God's still small voice. Stay close to God in daily prayer. In this way, when you are in His presence, you can tell God that you have faithfully served Him. In the end, you will be able to say I'm alright, and mean it.

What I once viewed as a devastating moment in my life, I know view as the fertile ground that made me the person I am today. Though the storms of my childhood I was forced to look at the dark side of my humanity. I was forced to look at my past not as a series of good and bad events, but rather events woven together to shape me, guide me toward my purpose. When I first started writing this book, I thought I should write about trauma in the African-American experience as related to our common past and how that past impacts how we deal with mental health today. While researching that I learned that my true purpose in writing this was to help that young child in many of us, who was forced to adapt to a set of terrifying events. I wanted to help that child, now an adult, to embrace new survival skills. We must acknowledge the importance of acquiring those skills. More importantly we must move toward our true source of strength: Jesus Christ.

Some of us may have used drugs, alcohol, self-mutilation, and even people along the way. It is only when we turn to God that our true healing can begin. Because we know He works all things for our good, we can utilize the many varieties of self-care, whether it is psychotherapy, yoga, or meditation. They all allow us to have a closer deeper relationship with Him. In doing so, we focus not on the shame of our past but on the gift of today. He has always walked with us, as He did with our ancestors. Carnal man would look at the brutality experienced by our ancestors as well as our own traumatic experience as evidence that God has forsaken us. That is a mistake that I have made myself.

The truth is He is with us in our misery. After all, He suffered the misery of the cross for us. In our misery he gives us a new song. How can I, a man of so many faults have a song in my heart? I have that song because God has given it to me. He also gives it to you. You see, He doesn't need perfect people. He needs broken people who recognize that they need a Savior. There is nothing grand in our lives in of itself. We become elevated by Him when we tell others about how great He is to us. I ask you to make use of all the treatment options available. Don't let your inner voice discourage you. Don't let others who don't understand your journey discourage you. Take the Lord's hand and let him guide you.

Your journey will most likely be different than mine but it will be just as rewarding. He will order your steps. He will bring people, books, social interactions and life experiences that will transform you. Stay in conversation with Him through your prayers. He will provide the resources you will need to heal. All these things provided by the Lord will help you to take the focus away from your inner thoughts of shame, guilt and anxiety and will help you focus on Him. His suffering for us on the cross was the ultimate sacrifice. He truly understands our pain. His wonderful love for us is truly amazing. Keep your heart and mind focused on Him and you will find your view of yourself changing for the better. It would be as if you woke up from a deep sleep. You will realize that the nightmare is over. Once you realize that, you will understand that you are alive in a way you have not been for years. The burden of shame and guilt has been washed away in your journey of recovery and you are now free to serve Him better.

After you enter this new stage of your life, embrace your truth. Face it head on. It will not be easy. You will come to an awareness of the extent of your pain. It may frighten you. You may, at times, feel you are alone. Realize that you are never alone for God is with you through it all. He will be the light within your soul. Let your light shine bright. Shine for your sake and for God's sake. Others will notice the change in you. They will ask you what caused it. Tell them, show them the way. No matter what path your journey takes you, He needs you to tell everyone how He has changed you.

You are not a victim, but a survivor of past events. You will find inner strength. God will provide you that strength. You are stronger than you think you are. He will help you move from surviving past events to enjoying the beauty of today. God will help you learn how to thrive as you cope with the pressures of day to day living. Trust in Him as He reveals your purpose. Know that life will continue to provide you with challenges. Instead of running from them, you will be able to boldly face them. You will then look to God to ask, what's next?

It's now your turn. Look back to the that young child within you before the abuse. The innocent child who was full of promise, that child filled with wonder. That child is still there inside of you. As a survivor of abuse, we often think we have no access to those memories. There is a conscious decision to suffer in silence. After all, who cares? We think what happened so many years ago is best forgotten. The truth is, as we try to put those memories out of our consciousness, a few threads persist. They are the tip of the emotional iceberg of our unconscious. That unconscious drives behaviors that create chaos in our lives. It causes the inability to maintain stable relationships, cause aberrant behavior and, in some, substance abuse. All because we choose not to discuss the events that has shaped our lives.

I wrote *I'm Alright* to reshape how childhood abuse survivors address their past. I think the first step is to not pretend what happened to us did not happen. But face the reality that it did. I told my story to encourage you to tell yours. Remember Romans 8:28, all things work together for your good. That is God's promise to you and me. I was encouraged to share my experiences by God to free me from the shame associated with it. I was not responsible for what happened to me as a child, but I am responsible for what I do with those experiences. I am responsible for all those I hurt. But God in His infinite wisdom has given me the ability to make amends. First, I had to realize that there was a problem that needed to be addressed. Then I realized that He would work it out for me through the various methods of treatment. They are available to you as well. But first you must look at that dark past, not in fear, but with the light of hope. I urge you to seek out a supportive community of abuse survivors.

I would love to see support groups of abuse survivors who all have the courage to share their experience, much like members of Alcoholics Anonymous and Narcotics Anonymous. Those communities share resources with each another, and engage in social activities together. It empowers each member based on their individual strengths. A group setting would remove the stigma associated trauma based on a shared experience.

I hope and pray that this book will start a dialogue among like-minded people. I extend my hand out to you metaphorically. Contact me on my website jamesgjones238.com and on Twitter @im_alright238.

AFTERWORD

My story began at a point of immense pain in my life. During that time, I described myself as Hurt Burt because my childhood innocence was shattered and I struggled to make sense of the senseless. Before then, I described myself as Newark Burt who represented a time in my life when I was a free spirit. A was child who lived through the social turmoil in Newark, New Jersey but I could hold my head up high as I enjoyed life. Newark Burt morphed into Hurt Burt. Hurt Burt became James who wore a mask of normalcy that over time developed multiple cracks. Eventually the mask was destroyed and revealed my fragility. This forced James, to change during the course this journey.

I recently had a conversation with my friend Ed Whitaker. Ed had always struggled with how to address me during our friendship. This is something that many people I meet at work who I later develop a personal relationship also struggled with. At work, everyone called me Dr. Jones, but in a social setting addressing me in that way was a bit formal. Ed, like many others simply called me James. Since Ed was familiar with my personal journey he suggested that I should now be known by a name that honors Newark Burt, Hurt Burt, James and Dr. Jones; all the parts of me, that existed somewhat separately. He decided, and I agree, that a new name would represent my awareness of this new phase of my life. He gave me the name DJ. I like it. DJ represents all of me as I stand in my truth.

It is truly amazing how God continues to work in my life. Ed chose to call me DJ. That name immediately resonated with me on a deep level. As Ed said it, that name felt and sounded right. As I prayed about that name God revealed to me and why that name was so important to me. DJ was the character in the movie *Promise* that I discussed earlier in the book. Ed of course was not aware of that movie. In the movie, DJ was a broken shell of a man who suffered with schizophrenia, but experienced a moment of joy. His experience resonates with me. I am DJ.

I first experienced joy as Newark Burt. I then surrendered the pursuit of joy to look for happiness as Hurt Burt and then James. I struggled to keep each part of me in their separate compartments. DJ represents the amalgam of them all. DJ realizes and accepts them all. DJ realizes that the cup is not half full as Hurt Burt would say, nor it is half empty as James would say. Instead he sees the cup as filled to overflowing. That is because it is filled with the love of Jesus. This overflowing of love is what propels DJ forward. It is what allows DJ to stand in his truth. As DJ, I must tell of God's love for us all.

I am reminded of a sermon given at the opening service of the annual revival at Enon Tabernacle Baptist Church called Eight Days of Glory, on October 15, 2016. The sermon was delivered by the inspirational and anointed Reverend Frederick Douglass Haynes III, Senior Pastor of Friendship West Baptist Church of Dallas, Texas. I look forward to hearing his sermon every year. I am never disappointed and this year was no different. His sermon was titled, "I Shook Up The World." In his sermon, Pastor Haynes talked about people being kept in the proverbial box and how they are told what to think by that box. The walls of the box say what won't happen and the ceiling of the box says what can't happen. Then he talked about an eagle that was well known to the people in a particular area. Someone shot the eagle in one of its wings with a BB gun. The eagle fell to the ground severely injured. There was a veterinarian and ornithologist, a person who studies birds, who saw the eagle fall. They nursed the bird back to health. After they released the eagle they noticed that it would fly at a height of ten feet and about forty-five feet before it fell back down to Earth. They examined the eagle and found that he was completely healed. They released the eagle again and again it fell back to earth after flying a short distance. The eagle had lost its confidence to fly even though he was healed. The bird could not move past its trauma.

That story resonated with me. What was even more amazing about it was the name of the eagle. His name was Burt. Before being shot Burt would soar high in the sky. Just like Newark Burt. After being shot down, for the eagle it was by a BB gun, for Hurt Burt it was trauma, he doubted his ability. Even with nurturing—for the eagle it was the veterinarian and ornithologist and me it was therapists and friends—Hurt Burt forgot how to soar. As Hurt Burt, I limited myself. I acted like I was still being traumatized. I don't know if the eagle ever learned to soar again, Pastor Haynes did not tell us. What I do know is that God did heal Hurt Burt. God transformed him into DJ and DJ is flying high.

On October 18, 2016 at 3:30 PM I had a strange sensation as I picked up a few items at the salad bar at the brand new Whole Foods Market located at 2101 Pennsylvania Avenue. I was impressed by the enormity of this multilevel superstore. I was enjoying myself as I was picking some lettuce for my salad. I felt a warm feeling in my chest and I notice a smile forming across my face. There was a sense of true joy that was different than what I felt in the past. It was just as intense, but there was a balanced quality to it. I was still very much aware of my relationship status and financial issues. What I noticed was that my trauma had faded to the background of the past where it belonged.

This wasn't like I not attending to my trauma, I was quite aware of it. It was simply in the past. It wasn't tapping into my self-esteem. I wasn't having my usual internal self-defeating internal monologue. Instead, I was basking in the moment. This was quite strange. You see, on many occasions, I was so haunted by memories of my trauma that I felt like I floated in a dissociative fog as if I was asleep. This time I was fully awake. No, better yet, I felt *alive*. I felt that I was my authentic self and for once I could fully accept myself.

I pray that this book inspires you to start your journey toward healing. There are so many treatment options available to you. I pray that through them, you will find your voice. Use that voice to speak your truth to people who are committed to your victory over the events in your past. I hope that my story will start a process where all abuse survivors can share their story with fellow abuse survivors first, and then with the world.

About the Author

James G. Jones, MD has practiced psychiatry for more than twenty years in Philadelphia, Pennsylvania. He was the Medical Director of the Crisis Response Center at Temple University, Episcopal Campus and an inpatient psychiatrist at the Girard Medical Center. He currently performs court ordered psychiatric evaluations at the Justice Juanita Kidd Stout Center of Criminal Justice. Dr. Jones also gives psychiatric evaluations to people with mental health and substance use disorders for Gaudenzia, Inc.

Born in Newark, New Jersey, Dr. Jones moved to Philadelphia, Pennsylvania with his siblings shortly after the Newark riots of the summer 1967. He was raised in a household where emotional and physical abuse were the norm. Despite this, he could achieve academically, though he struggled with self-esteem issues and low level depression throughout his life. He became a Christian as a young adult, yet still struggled with his faith. He was involved in therapy on several occasions throughout his life with very little success. In 2014, a movie triggered his first flashback. This event set into motion his desire to understand his traumatic past and the treatment options available. In this pursuit, he found his Christian faith deepening. As a result, he was inspired to write *I'm Alright*. Its purpose is to chronicle his journey in the context of his ancestry and Christian faith to inspire other to begin their own.

The Logo

You may wonder how I developed the logo for this book. It was the culmination of several ideas that came together all at once. I wanted a boldface font with soft curves. I wanted that font to be outlined so that it would stand out. I listened to the lyrics of a song by Natalie Grant called "Clean." The words of the song spoke to me. They inspired me to redesign the font with graphic elements.

I was first inspired by my Senior Pastor Dr. Alyn E. Waller of Enon Tabernacle Baptist Church. During one of his magnificent sermon he talked about kintsugi. Kintsugi is Japanese pottery that has been broken and subsequently fixed with silver, gold or platinum. In performing this kind of repair, it looks at the damage as a part of the pottery's history. Its repair serves to highlight that it has been damaged and repaired with a metal far more valuable than the original pottery itself. The kintsugi pottery is a metaphor for how we become valuable to God by allowing Him to fix our brokenness.

I thought of Isaiah 64:8 (KJV) "But thou art our Father: we are the clay, and thou our potter: and we all are the work of thy hand" and Jeremiah 18:6b (KJV)" ...Behold, as the clay is in the potter's hand, so are ye in mine hand, O house of Israel." I envision the letters of the font in the beginning to represent pottery that the Lord is "repairing" in a different way. Just as in kintsugi, the repair God makes is made with the gold of His eternal love. The "i" in alright represents you kneeling praying to God accepting Christ, believing that He died for your sins and mine. By confessing that He is your Lord and Savior and you become as white as snow. You represent His purity. The cracks in your "pottery," which represent your life, slowly fade away as you move to the letter "t" and you see you have been made whole by Christ.

Resources

The Holy Bible
The Battlefield of the Mind by Joyce Meyer
The Body Keeps the Score by Bessel Van der Kolk, MD
Christian Meditation by James Finley
Contemplative Prayer by Thomas Merton
The EMDR Revolution: Change Your Life One Memory At A Time by Tal Croitoru
The Emotionally Abusive Relationship by Beverly Engel
Frederick Douglass: My Bondage and My Freedom by Dr. James M'Cune Smith
The Fear Cure by Lissa Rankin
Forgiving Our Fathers and Mothers by Jill Hubbard, Leslie Leyland Fields
Forgiveness by Iyanla Vanzant
Getting Past Your Past by Francine Shapiro, PhD
In Our Own Voice by Vanessa Jackson, LCSW
It Wasn't Your Fault by Beverly Engel
Jung by Anthony Stevens
Love Yourself Like Your Life Depends On It by Kamal Ravikant
Mere Christianity by C.S. Lewis
The Mind-Body Code by Dr. Mario Martinez
The Protest Psychosis by Jonathan M. Metzl MD, PhD.
Post Traumatic Slave Syndrome by Joy DeGruy, PhD.
Soul Detox by Craig Groeschel
Trauma and Recovery by Judith Lewis Herman, MD

The Trauma Zone: Trusting God for Emotional Healing by R. Dandridge Collins
Trusting God by Jerry Bridges

Made in the USA
Middletown, DE
31 March 2017